THE COMPLETE ZERO POINT RECIPES FOR WEIGHT LOSS

Maximum Results: Your Comprehensive Guide to Weight Loss Success

Dr. Melissa R. Steven

INTRODUCTION

Welcome to "The Complete Zero Point Recipes for Weight Loss" – your ultimate guide to harnessing the power of zero point foods to achieve your health and wellness goals. In a world where fad diets and quick-fix solutions abound, the concept of zero point recipes offers a refreshing and sustainable approach to weight loss.

At the heart of this book lies the understanding that not all calories are created equal. Zero point foods, as defined by various dietary programs such as Weight Watchers, are nutrient-dense, low-calorie options that you can enjoy in abundance without worrying about tipping the scales. These foods are not just about filling your plate; they are about nourishing your body and satisfying your cravings while promoting a sense of fullness and satisfaction.

In this comprehensive guide, we will delve deep into the world of zero point cooking, exploring the myriad of ingredients and flavors that can transform your meals from bland to extraordinary. From energizing breakfasts to satisfying main courses, from refreshing salads to decadent desserts – we've got you covered with a wide array of recipes that will tantalize your taste buds and keep you on track towards your weight loss goals.

However, this book is not merely a compilation of recipes. It's a roadmap for success, providing you with the tools, tips, and strategies you need to make zero point eating a sustainable lifestyle choice. Whether you're a seasoned cook or a kitchen novice, whether you're embarking on your weight loss journey for the first time or looking for fresh inspiration to reignite your progress, this book is designed to empower you every step of the way.

So, if you're ready to say goodbye to restrictive diets and calorie counting and hello to delicious, nutritious meals that will nourish your body and fuel your weight loss journey, then let's dive in together. "The Complete Zero Point Recipes for Weight Loss" is not just a cookbook – it's your ticket to a healthier, happier you.

Let's get cooking!

TABLE OF CONTENTS

I. Understanding Zero Point Foods and Weight Loss

In the realm of weight loss and dietary management, the concept of zero point foods has gained significant traction in recent years. Originating from programs like Weight Watchers, zero point foods refer to a specific category of foods that are designated as having zero or very low points in their respective systems. While the exact list of zero point foods may vary depending on the program, they generally include fruits, vegetables, lean proteins, and certain other nutritious options.

1 The Role of Zero Point Foods

Zero point foods play a pivotal role in weight loss for several reasons. Firstly, they are typically low in calories, making them ideal choices for individuals looking to reduce their overall calorie intake without sacrificing volume or satiety. By incorporating these foods into your meals and snacks, you can create a sense of fullness and satisfaction without consuming excess calories.

Moreover, zero point foods are often rich in essential nutrients such as vitamins, minerals, and fiber. This means that not only do they contribute to your overall health and well-being, but they also help to support your body's various physiological functions. Fiber, in particular, is renowned for its role in promoting digestive health, regulating blood sugar levels, and aiding in weight management by promoting feelings of fullness and preventing overeating.

2 Understanding the Zero Point System

It's important to note that the designation of zero points does not mean that these foods have zero calories or should be consumed in unlimited quantities. Rather, it reflects the fact that these foods are deemed to be less likely to contribute to weight gain when consumed in moderation. Portion control and mindful eating remain essential components of any successful weight loss journey, even when focusing on zero point foods.

Additionally, while zero point foods can certainly form the foundation of a healthy diet, they should ideally be combined with a diverse range of other nutrient-dense foods to ensure that your body receives all the essential nutrients it needs for optimal functioning. Balancing zero point foods with sources of healthy fats, whole grains, and lean proteins can help to create a well-rounded and sustainable eating plan.

3 Harnessing the Power of Zero Point Foods

Incorporating zero point foods into your diet can be a game-changer when it comes to achieving your weight loss goals. Not only do they provide a wealth of nutritional benefits, but they also offer versatility and flexibility in meal planning. From colorful salads and hearty soups to satisfying stir-fries and delicious fruit smoothies, the possibilities for incorporating zero point foods into your meals are endless.

By understanding the role of zero point foods and learning how to incorporate them into your daily eating habits, you can take a significant step towards achieving sustainable weight loss and improved overall health. In the chapters that follow, we will explore a variety of delicious recipes and meal ideas that showcase the versatility and flavor of zero point foods, helping you to create meals that are both nutritious and satisfying.

Chapter 1: The Power of Zero Point Foods

1.1 Exploring Zero Point Foods and Their Role in Weight Loss

Zero point foods are a cornerstone of many successful weight loss programs, offering individuals a variety of nutritious options that can be enjoyed without the need for extensive calorie counting or portion control. Understanding the nature of these foods and their impact on weight loss is essential for anyone looking to adopt a healthier lifestyle and shed unwanted pounds.

What are Zero Point Foods?

Zero point foods, as the name suggests, are foods that are assigned zero or very low point values in certain weight loss programs, such as Weight Watchers. These foods are typically low in calories and rich in essential nutrients, making them ideal choices for individuals looking to lose weight without feeling deprived or hungry.

Zero Point Foods' Significance in Weight Loss

One of the key advantages of zero point foods is their ability to help individuals feel satisfied and full while consuming fewer calories. Many zero point foods, such as fruits and vegetables, are high in water and fiber, both of which contribute to a feeling of satiety and can help prevent overeating.

By incorporating zero point foods into meals and snacks, individuals can increase the volume of their food intake without significantly increasing their calorie intake. This can lead to a reduced overall calorie intake, which is essential for weight loss.

The Advantages of Zero Point Foods for Nutrition

In addition to their low calorie content, zero point foods are often packed with essential nutrients that are important for overall health and well-being. Fruits and vegetables, for example, are rich in vitamins, minerals, and antioxidants that support immune function, promote healthy digestion, and reduce the risk of chronic diseases such as heart disease and cancer.

Lean proteins, another category of zero point foods, are essential for muscle repair and growth, as well as for maintaining a healthy metabolism. Including lean proteins such as chicken, turkey, fish, and tofu in your diet can help you feel full and satisfied while supporting your weight loss efforts.

Including Foods With No Points in Your Diet

One of the key benefits of zero point foods is their versatility and flexibility in meal planning. From colorful salads and hearty soups to flavorful stir-fries and satisfying snacks, there are countless ways to incorporate zero point foods into your daily meals and snacks.

Experimenting with different recipes and cooking methods can help keep meals exciting and enjoyable, preventing boredom and reducing the likelihood of falling off track with your weight loss goals. Additionally, focusing on whole, minimally processed foods can help ensure that you're getting the most nutritional value out of your meals.

In the following chapters, we'll explore a variety of delicious recipes and meal ideas that showcase the versatility and flavor of zero point foods. Whether you're a seasoned chef or a novice cook, there's something for everyone to enjoy as we embark on this journey towards healthier eating and sustainable weight loss.

1.2 How Zero Point Foods Can Revolutionize Your Eating Habits

The concept of zero point foods offers a refreshing and sustainable approach to revolutionizing your eating habits. By embracing the abundance of nutritious and satisfying options available among zero point foods, you can transform your relationship with food and pave the way for long-term health and wellness.

Freedom from Restriction

One of the most liberating aspects of zero point foods is the freedom they provide from the constraints of traditional dieting. Rather than focusing on deprivation and strict calorie counting, zero point foods allow you to eat until you're satisfied without worrying about exceeding your daily allotment of points or calories.

This newfound sense of freedom can be incredibly empowering, enabling you to listen to your body's hunger and fullness cues and eat in a way that feels natural and intuitive. Gone are the days of feeling guilty or ashamed for indulging in your favorite foods – with zero point foods, you can enjoy a wide variety of delicious options without fear of derailing your progress.

Embracing Nutrient-Dense Choices

Zero point foods are not just about filling your plate; they're about nourishing your body with nutrient-dense ingredients that support your overall health and well-being. Fruits and vegetables, for example, are rich in vitamins, minerals, and antioxidants that play essential roles in everything from immune function to cellular repair.

By incorporating more zero point foods into your diet, you can increase your intake of these essential nutrients while reducing your consumption of less nutritious options. This shift towards a more nutrient-dense eating pattern can have profound effects on your energy levels, mood, and overall vitality, setting you up for success both in the short and long term.

Building Sustainable Habits

Perhaps the most significant way that zero point foods can revolutionize your eating habits is by helping you build sustainable, lifelong habits that support your health and wellness goals. Unlike restrictive diets that are difficult to maintain over time, zero point foods offer a flexible and adaptable framework that can be tailored to fit your individual preferences and lifestyle.

By learning to incorporate more zero point foods into your meals and snacks, you can develop healthier eating habits that last a lifetime. This might mean swapping out high-calorie snacks for crunchy vegetables or experimenting with new recipes that feature lean proteins and vibrant produce. Whatever approach you choose, the key is to focus on balance, variety, and moderation, ensuring that you're nourishing your body while still enjoying the foods you love.

Chapter 2: Getting Started with Zero Point Cooking

2.1 Essential Ingredients and Tools for Zero Point Cooking

Embarking on a journey of zero point cooking opens up a world of possibilities for creating delicious, nutritious meals that support your weight loss goals. To make the most of this culinary adventure, it's essential to have the right ingredients and tools on hand to help you prepare flavorful dishes with ease and efficiency.

Stocking Your Pantry

Building a well-stocked pantry is the first step towards successful zero point cooking. By keeping a variety of staple ingredients on hand, you'll always have the foundation for creating satisfying meals without the need for last-minute trips to the grocery store. Some essential pantry items for zero point cooking include:

- Herbs and Spices: Herbs and spices are the secret weapons of zero point cooking, adding flavor and depth to dishes without adding extra calories. Keep a variety of dried herbs and spices on hand, such as oregano, basil, cumin, paprika, and garlic powder, to enhance the taste of your meals.

- Low-Sodium Broths and Stocks: Broths and stocks are versatile ingredients that can be used as a base for soups, stews, and sauces. Opt for low-sodium varieties to control the salt content of your dishes while still adding rich, savory flavor.

- Canned Tomatoes: Canned tomatoes are a pantry staple that can be used to create a wide range of dishes, from hearty pasta sauces to flavorful curries. Look for canned tomatoes with no added salt or sugar to keep your recipes as healthy as possible.

- Whole Grains: Whole grains such as brown rice, quinoa, and barley are nutritious, filling ingredients that can be used as a base for grain bowls, salads, and side dishes. Keep a variety of whole grains on hand to add texture and substance to your meals.

- Legumes: Beans, lentils, and chickpeas are excellent sources of protein and fiber, making them ideal ingredients for zero point cooking. Stock up on canned or dried legumes to incorporate into soups, stews, salads, and more.

Equipping Your Kitchen

In addition to stocking your pantry with essential ingredients, it's also important to have the right tools and equipment to support your zero point cooking endeavors. While you don't need a fancy kitchen setup to create delicious meals, having a few key items on hand can make the cooking process easier and more enjoyable. Some essential tools for zero point cooking include:

- Sharp Knives: A good set of sharp knives is essential for prepping ingredients quickly and safely. Invest in a chef's knife, paring knife, and serrated knife to cover all your cutting needs.

- Cutting Boards: Multiple cutting boards in different sizes are handy for chopping vegetables, fruits, and herbs without cross-contamination. Opt for cutting boards made of wood or plastic that are easy to clean and maintain.

- Non-Stick Cookware: Non-stick pots and pans are ideal for zero point cooking, as they require less oil and fat to prevent sticking. Invest in a high-quality non-stick skillet, saucepan, and stockpot to cover all your cooking needs.

- Steamer Basket: A steamer basket is a versatile tool that allows you to cook vegetables, seafood, and grains quickly and healthily. Look for a steamer basket that fits securely in your pots and pans and is easy to clean.

- Blender or Food Processor: A blender or food processor is essential for creating smoothies, sauces, dips, and purees. Choose a high-powered blender or food processor that can handle a variety of ingredients and textures with ease.

By stocking your pantry with essential ingredients and equipping your kitchen with the right tools, you'll be well-prepared to embark on your zero point cooking journey with confidence and creativity. With a little planning and preparation, you can enjoy delicious, nutritious meals that support your weight loss goals and satisfy your taste buds.

2.2 Tips for Meal Planning with Zero Point Foods

Effective meal planning is the cornerstone of successful weight loss and healthy eating habits, and incorporating zero point foods into your meal plans can help streamline the process while maximizing flavor and nutrition. By following these tips for meal planning with zero point foods, you can simplify your cooking routine, stay on track with your weight loss goals, and enjoy delicious, satisfying meals every day.

1. Start with a Weekly Meal Plan

Begin your meal planning process by creating a weekly meal plan that outlines the main meals and snacks you'll be enjoying throughout the week. Take into account your schedule, preferences, and any special occasions or events that may impact your meal choices. Having a clear plan in place can help you stay organized and motivated, making it easier to stick to your healthy eating goals.

2. Focus on Variety and Balance

When planning your meals, aim to incorporate a variety of zero point foods to ensure you're getting a wide range of nutrients and flavors. Include plenty of colorful fruits and vegetables, lean proteins, whole grains, and legumes to create balanced, satisfying meals that keep you feeling full and energized throughout the day.

3. Mix and Match Flavors and Textures

Get creative with your meal planning by experimenting with different flavor profiles, textures, and cooking techniques. Mix and match ingredients to create interesting and satisfying combinations, such as pairing sweet fruits with savory proteins or adding crunchy vegetables to creamy soups. Don't be afraid to try new recipes and flavor combinations – you may discover new favorite dishes along the way!

4. Prep Ingredients in Advance

Save time and energy during the week by prepping ingredients in advance whenever possible. Wash, chop, and portion out fruits and vegetables, cook grains and legumes, and marinate proteins ahead of time to streamline the cooking process and make mealtime preparation a breeze. Store prepped ingredients in airtight containers in the fridge for easy access throughout the week.

5. Use Zero Point Foods as Meal Fillers

Zero point foods can serve as excellent meal fillers, adding volume and texture to dishes without adding extra calories. Incorporate plenty of leafy greens, non-starchy vegetables, and low-calorie fruits into your meals to bulk them up and increase their satiety factor. This can help you feel fuller for longer and reduce the temptation to overeat.

6. Don't Forget About Portion Control

While zero point foods can be enjoyed in abundance, it's still important to practice portion control to avoid overeating. Pay attention to serving sizes and be mindful of your hunger and fullness cues when enjoying zero point meals and snacks. Eating slowly, savoring each bite, and stopping when you feel satisfied can help prevent unnecessary calorie consumption.

7. Plan for Flexibility

Finally, remember that meal planning with zero point foods should be flexible and adaptable to your individual needs and preferences. Don't feel constrained by rigid meal plans – allow yourself the freedom to make changes and adjustments as needed based on how you're feeling and what ingredients you have on hand. The goal is to create a sustainable eating plan that works for you in the long term.

By following these tips for meal planning with zero point foods, you can simplify your cooking routine, maximize flavor and nutrition, and stay on track with your weight loss goals. With a little planning and creativity, you can enjoy delicious, satisfying meals that support your health and well-being every day.

Chapter 3: Breakfasts to Jumpstart Your Day

3.1 Energizing Zero Point Breakfast Smoothies

1. Berry Blast Breakfast Smoothie

Ingredients:

- 1 cup unsweetened almond milk
- 1/2 cup plain non-fat Greek yogurt
- 1/2 cup frozen mixed berries (such as strawberries, blueberries, and raspberries)
- 1/2 frozen banana
- 1 tablespoon ground flaxseed
- Optional: 1 teaspoon honey or maple syrup for added sweetness

Directions:

1. In a blender, combine all ingredients.
2. Blend till creamy and smooth.
3. Transfer into glasses and serve right away.

Servings: 1

Nutritional Information (per serving):

Calories: 180 kcal

Total Fat: 4g

Saturated Fat: 0.3g

Trans Fat: 0g

Cholesterol: 0mg

Sodium: 120mg

Total Carbohydrates: 28g

Dietary Fiber: 6g

Sugars: 15g

Protein: 12g

2. Green Power Smoothie

Ingredients:

- 1 cup unsweetened almond milk
- 1/2 cup plain non-fat Greek yogurt
- 1/2 frozen banana
- 1/2 cup frozen mango chunks
- 1 cup fresh spinach
- 1 tablespoon chia seeds
- Optional: squeeze of fresh lime juice

Directions:

1. Fill a blender with all the ingredients.
2. Blend till creamy and smooth.
3. After pouring into a glass, savor!

Servings: 1

Nutritional Information (per serving):

Calories: 220 kcal

Total Fat: 5g

Saturated Fat: 0.4g

Trans Fat: 0g

Cholesterol: 0mg

Sodium: 140mg

Total Carbohydrates: 35g

Dietary Fiber: 8g

Sugars: 18g

Protein: 13g

3. Tropical Paradise Smoothie

Ingredients:

- 1 cup unsweetened coconut milk
- 1/2 cup plain non-fat Greek yogurt
- 1/2 frozen banana
- 1/2 cup frozen pineapple chunks
- 1/2 cup frozen mango chunks
- 1 tablespoon shredded coconut

Directions:

1. Combine all ingredients in a blender.
2. Blend until smooth and creamy.
3. Pour into glasses and serve immediately.

Servings: 1

Nutritional Information (per serving):

Calories: 240 kcal

Total Fat: 6g

Saturated Fat: 3g

Trans Fat: 0g

Cholesterol: 0mg

Sodium: 130mg

Total Carbohydrates: 38g

Dietary Fiber: 6g

Sugars: 24g

Protein: 14g

4. Peanut Butter Banana Smoothie

Ingredients:

- 1 cup unsweetened almond milk
- 1/2 cup plain non-fat Greek yogurt
- 1/2 frozen banana
- 2 tablespoons natural peanut butter
- 1 tablespoon cocoa powder
- Optional: 1 teaspoon honey or maple syrup for added sweetness

Directions:

1. Blend all ingredients in a blender until smooth.
2. Adjust sweetness if necessary.
3. Pour into a glass and enjoy!

Servings: 1

Nutritional Information (per serving):

Calories: 320 kcal

Total Fat: 18g

Saturated Fat: 2.5g

Trans Fat: 0g

Cholesterol: 0mg

Sodium: 220mg

Total Carbohydrates: 26g

Dietary Fiber: 6g

Sugars: 11g

Protein: 20g

5. Protein-Packed Berry Smoothie

Ingredients:

- 1 cup unsweetened almond milk
- 1/2 cup plain non-fat Greek yogurt
- 1/2 cup frozen mixed berries (such as strawberries, blueberries, and raspberries)
- 1 scoop vanilla protein powder
- 1 tablespoon chia seeds

Directions:

1. Combine all ingredients in a blender.
2. Blend until smooth and creamy.
3. Pour into glasses and serve immediately.

Servings: 1

Nutritional Information (per serving):

Calories: 220 kcal

Total Fat: 5g

Saturated Fat: 0.3g

Trans Fat: 0g

Cholesterol: 0mg

Sodium: 150mg

Total Carbohydrates: 20g

Dietary Fiber: 7g

Sugars: 8g

Protein: 25g

Adjust ingredients and servings as needed to fit your personal dietary preferences and requirements. Enjoy these energizing zero point breakfast smoothies as part of a balanced and nutritious meal!

3.2 Flavorful Egg-Free Breakfast Bowls

1. Berry Bliss Breakfast Bowl

Ingredients:

- 1/2 cup rolled oats
- One cup unsweetened almond milk
- 1/2 cup mixed berries (such as strawberries, blueberries, and raspberries)
- 1 tablespoon chia seeds
- 1 tablespoon almond butter
- Optional toppings: sliced banana, shredded coconut, chopped nuts

Directions:

1. Place the almond milk and rolled oats in a saucepan.
2. Cook over medium heat, stirring occasionally, until the oats are creamy and tender, about 5-7 minutes.
3. Transfer the cooked oats to a bowl and top with mixed berries, chia seeds, and almond butter.
4. Add any optional toppings as desired.
5. Serve warm and enjoy!

Servings: 1

Nutritional Information (per serving):

Calories: 350 kcal

Total Fat: 14g

Saturated Fat: 1g

Trans Fat: 0g

Cholesterol: 0mg

Sodium: 170mg

Total Carbohydrates: 48g

Dietary Fiber: 11g

Sugars: 10g

Protein: 10g

2. Tropical Paradise Breakfast Bowl

Ingredients:

- 1/2 cup cooked quinoa
- 1/2 cup unsweetened coconut milk
- 1/2 cup diced mango
- 1/4 cup diced pineapple
- 1 tablespoon shredded coconut
- One tablespoon chopped macadamia nuts
- Optional toppings: sliced banana, kiwi, passion fruit

Directions:

1. In a bowl, combine the cooked quinoa and coconut milk.
2. Top with diced mango, pineapple, shredded coconut, and chopped macadamia nuts.
3. Add any optional toppings as desired.
4. Serve either at room temperature or cold.

Servings: 1

Nutritional Information (per serving):

Calories: 380 kcal

Total Fat: 18g

Saturated Fat: 8g

Trans Fat: 0g

Cholesterol: 0mg

Sodium: 20mg

Total Carbohydrates: 52g

Dietary Fiber: 7g

Sugars: 23g

Protein: 7g

3. Protein-Packed Peanut Butter Breakfast Bowl

Ingredients:

- 1/2 cup plain non-fat Greek yogurt
- 1/4 cup rolled oats
- 1 tablespoon natural peanut butter
- 1/2 banana, sliced
- One spoonful of maple syrup or honey
- Optional toppings: sliced strawberries, granola, chocolate chips

Directions:

1. In a bowl, combine the Greek yogurt, rolled oats, and peanut butter.
2. Blend thoroughly until everything is properly integrated.
3. Top with sliced banana and drizzle with honey or maple syrup.
4. Add any optional toppings as desired.
5. Serve chilled or at room temperature.

Servings: 1

Nutritional Information (per serving):

Calories: 380 kcal

Total Fat: 12g

Saturated Fat: 2g

Trans Fat: 0g

Cholesterol: 5mg

Sodium: 70mg

Total Carbohydrates: 50g

Dietary Fiber: 5g

Sugars: 29g

Protein: 20g

4. Acai Berry Breakfast Bowl

Ingredients:

- One frozen acai packet without sugar
- 1/2 cup unsweetened almond milk
- 1/2 banana, sliced
- 1/4 cup granola
- 1 tablespoon chia seeds
- Optional toppings: sliced strawberries, blueberries, coconut flakes

Directions:

1. In a blender, combine the frozen acai packet and almond milk.
2. Blend till creamy and smooth.
3. Transfer the acai blend into a bowl.
4. Top with sliced banana, granola, and chia seeds.
5. Add any optional toppings as desired.
6. Serve immediately and enjoy!

Servings: 1

Nutritional Information (per serving):

Calories: 320 kcal

Total Fat: 12g

Saturated Fat: 2g

Trans Fat: 0g

Cholesterol: 0mg

Sodium: 70mg

Total Carbohydrates: 48g

Dietary Fiber: 10g

Sugars: 22g

Protein: 7g

5. Chocolate Banana Breakfast Bowl

Ingredients:

- 1/2 cup unsweetened almond milk
- 1/4 cup rolled oats
- 1 tablespoon cocoa powder
- 1/2 banana, sliced
- 1 tablespoon almond butter
- Optional toppings: sliced strawberries, shredded coconut, chocolate chips

Directions:

1. In a saucepan, combine the almond milk, rolled oats, and cocoa powder.
2. Cook over medium heat, stirring occasionally, until the oats are creamy and tender, about 5-7 minutes.
3. Transfer the cooked oats to a bowl.
4. Top with sliced banana and almond butter.
5. Add any optional toppings as desired.
6. Serve warm and enjoy!

Servings: 1

Nutritional Information (per serving):

Calories: 330 kcal
Total Fat: 12g
Saturated Fat: 2g
Trans Fat: 0g
Cholesterol: 0mg
Sodium: 100mg
Total Carbohydrates: 50g
Dietary Fiber: 8g

Sugars: 17g
Protein: 9g

Adjust ingredients and servings as needed to fit your personal dietary preferences and requirements. Enjoy these flavorful egg-free breakfast bowls as part of a balanced and nutritious meal!

3.3 Creative Pancake and Waffle Alternatives

1. Banana Oat Pancakes

Ingredients:

- 1 ripe banana
- 1/2 cup rolled oats
- 1/4 cup unsweetened almond milk
- 1 teaspoon baking powder
- 1/2 teaspoon cinnamon
- Optional toppings: fresh berries, sliced bananas, maple syrup

Directions:

1. In a blender or food processor, combine the ripe banana, rolled oats, almond milk, baking powder, and cinnamon.
2. Blend until smooth and creamy, adding more almond milk if needed to achieve the desired consistency.
3. Over medium heat, preheat a nonstick skillet or griddle.
4. Transfer 1/4 cup of the pancake mixture to the skillet and let it cook for two to three minutes, or until bubbles start to appear on the top.
5. After flipping, cook the pancake for a further one to two minutes, or until golden brown.
6. Proceed with the leftover batter.
7. Warm pancakes should be served with your preferred toppings.
8. Servings: 2 (makes about 4 medium-sized pancakes)

Nutritional Information (per serving):

Calories: 190 kcal

Total Fat: 2g

Saturated Fat: 0g

Trans Fat: 0g

Cholesterol: 0mg

Sodium: 190mg

Total Carbohydrates: 42g

Dietary Fiber: 5g

Sugars: 13g

Protein: 5g

2. Sweet Potato Waffles

Ingredients:

- 1 cup cooked and mashed sweet potato
- 1/2 cup almond flour
- 2 eggs
- 1 teaspoon baking powder
- 1/2 teaspoon cinnamon
- Pinch of salt
- Optional toppings: Greek yogurt, sliced almonds, honey

Directions:

1. In a mixing bowl, combine the mashed sweet potato, almond flour, eggs, baking powder, cinnamon, and salt.
2. Stir until well combined.
3. As directed by the manufacturer, preheat your waffle iron.
4. Spray cooking spray on the waffle iron very lightly.
5. Evenly distribute the sweet potato batter using a spoon onto the waffle iron.
6. Close the waffle iron and cook for 5 to 7 minutes, or until the waffles are crisp and golden brown.
7. Proceed with the leftover batter.
8. Warm waffles should be served with your preferred toppings.
9. Servings: 2 (makes about 4 small waffles)

Nutritional Information (per serving):

Calories: 240 kcal

Total Fat: 13g

Saturated Fat: 1.5g

Trans Fat: 0g

Cholesterol: 106mg

Sodium: 320mg

Total Carbohydrates: 22g

Dietary Fiber: 4g

Sugars: 5g

Protein: 10g

3. Coconut Flour Pancakes

Ingredients:

- 1/4 cup coconut flour
- 2 eggs
- 1/2 cup unsweetened almond milk
- 1 tablespoon maple syrup
- 1 teaspoon baking powder
- 1/2 teaspoon vanilla extract
- Pinch of salt
- Optional toppings: fresh fruit, coconut flakes, honey

Directions:

1. In a mixing bowl, whisk together the coconut flour, eggs, almond milk, maple syrup, baking powder, vanilla extract, and salt until smooth.
2. To let the coconut flour absorb the liquid, let the batter sit for a few minutes.
3. Over medium heat, preheat a nonstick skillet or griddle.
4. For each pancake, place one to two teaspoons of the batter onto the griddle.

5. Cook for a further one to two minutes, or until golden brown, after flipping when bubbles start to appear on the surface.

6. Repeat with the remaining batter.

7. Serve the pancakes warm with your favorite toppings.

8. Servings: 2 (makes about 6 small pancakes)

Nutritional Information (per serving):

Calories: 160 kcal

Total Fat: 7g

Saturated Fat: 2g

Trans Fat: 0g

Cholesterol: 186mg

Sodium: 370mg

Total Carbohydrates: 15g

Dietary Fiber: 5g

Sugars: 6g

Protein: 9g

4. Zucchini Waffles

Ingredients:

- 1 cup shredded zucchini, excess moisture squeezed out
- 1/2 cup almond flour
- 2 eggs
- 1/2 teaspoon baking powder
- 1/2 teaspoon garlic powder
- Salt and pepper to taste
- Optional toppings: Greek yogurt, sliced tomatoes, avocado slices

Directions:

1. In a mixing bowl, combine the shredded zucchini, almond flour, eggs, baking powder, garlic powder, salt, and pepper.
2. Stir until well combined.
3. Preheat your waffle iron according to the manufacturer's instructions.
4. Lightly grease the waffle iron with cooking spray.
5. Spoon the zucchini batter onto the waffle iron and spread it out evenly.
6. Close the waffle iron and cook until the waffles are golden brown and crisp, about 5-7 minutes.
7. Repeat with the remaining batter.
8. Serve the waffles warm with your favorite toppings.
9. Servings: 2 (makes about 4 small waffles)

Nutritional Information (per serving):

Calories: 190 kcal
Total Fat: 14g
Saturated Fat: 1.5g
Trans Fat: 0g
Cholesterol: 106mg
Sodium: 150mg
Total Carbohydrates: 9g
Dietary Fiber: 3g
Sugars: 3g
Protein: 9g

5. Cauliflower Pancakes

Ingredients:

- 1 cup riced cauliflower, cooked and cooled
- 2 eggs

- 1/4 cup almond flour
- 1/4 cup shredded cheddar cheese
- 1/4 teaspoon garlic powder
- Salt and pepper to taste
- Optional toppings: Greek yogurt, salsa, sliced avocado

Directions:

1. In a mixing bowl, combine the riced cauliflower, eggs, almond flour, shredded cheddar cheese, garlic powder, salt, and pepper.
2. Stir until well combined.
3. Heat a non-stick skillet or griddle over medium heat.
4. Spoon 1-2 tablespoons of the pancake batter onto the skillet for each pancake.
5. Cook until golden brown on the bottom, then flip and cook for an additional 1-2 minutes, until cooked through and crispy.
6. Repeat with the remaining batter.
7. Serve the pancakes warm with your favorite toppings.
8. Servings: 2 (makes about 6 small pancakes)

Nutritional Information (per serving):

Calories: 190 kcal

Total Fat: 12g

Saturated Fat: 4g

Trans Fat: 0g

Cholesterol: 106mg

Sodium: 220mg

Total Carbohydrates: 9g

Dietary Fiber: 3g

Sugars: 3g

Protein: 11g

Adjust ingredients and servings as needed to fit your personal dietary preferences and requirements. Enjoy these creative pancake and waffle alternatives as part of a delicious and nutritious breakfast!

Chapter 4: Satisfying Soups and Salads

4.1 Hearty Vegetable Soups for Nourishment

1. Classic Minestrone Soup

Ingredients:

- 1 tablespoon olive oil
- 1 onion, diced
- 2 cloves garlic, minced
- 2 carrots, diced
- 2 celery stalks, diced
- 1 zucchini, diced
- 1 cup green beans, chopped
- 1 can (14 oz) diced tomatoes
- 6 cups vegetable broth
- One can (15 oz) of washed and drained kidney beans
- 1 cup small pasta (such as ditalini or small shells)
- 1 teaspoon dried basil
- 1 teaspoon dried oregano
- Salt and pepper to taste
- Grated Parmesan cheese for serving (optional)

Directions:

1. In a big saucepan, warm the olive oil over medium heat. Add the onion and garlic, and sauté until softened, about 5 minutes.
2. Add the carrots, celery, zucchini, and green beans to the pot. Cook for another 5 minutes, until the vegetables begin to soften.
3. Stir in the diced tomatoes, vegetable broth, kidney beans, pasta, basil, and oregano. Bring the soup to a simmer.
4. Cook for 10-15 minutes, until the pasta and vegetables are tender.

5. Add salt and pepper to taste when preparing the soup.

6. If preferred, top warm dishes with grated Parmesan cheese.

Servings: 6

Nutritional Information (per serving):

Calories: 220 kcal

Total Fat: 3g

Saturated Fat: 0.5g

Trans Fat: 0g

Cholesterol: 0mg

Sodium: 780mg

Total Carbohydrates: 42g

Dietary Fiber: 10g

Sugars: 8g

Protein: 9g

2. Lentil Vegetable Soup

Ingredients:

- 1 tablespoon olive oil
- 1 onion, diced
- 2 carrots, diced
- 2 celery stalks, diced
- 2 cloves garlic, minced
- 1 cup dried green lentils, rinsed
- 6 cups vegetable broth
- 1 can (14 oz) diced tomatoes
- 1 teaspoon ground cumin
- 1 teaspoon paprika
- Salt and pepper to taste
- For garnish, use fresh parsley (optional).

Directions:

1. Add the onion, carrots, and celery and sauté for approximately 5 minutes, or until the vegetables soften.
2. Garlic is added to the saucepan and cooked for an additional minute.
3. Add the diced tomatoes, vegetable broth, paprika, cumin, and dry lentils and stir. Simmer the soup for a while.
4. Cook until the lentils are cooked, 20 to 25 minutes.
5. If preferred, top hot dish with fresh parsley.5 g

Servings: 6

Nutritional Information (per serving):

Calories: 220 kcal
Total Fat: 3g
Saturated Fat: 0.5g
Trans Fat: 0g
Cholesterol: 0mg
Sodium: 760mg
Total Carbohydrates: 37g
Dietary Fiber: 12g
Sugars: 7g
Protein: 12g

3. Chunky Vegetable Barley Soup

Ingredients:

- 1 tablespoon olive oil
- 1 onion, diced
- 2 carrots, diced

- 2 celery stalks, diced
- 2 cloves garlic, minced
- 1 cup pearl barley
- 6 cups vegetable broth
- 1 can (14 oz) diced tomatoes
- 1 teaspoon dried thyme
- 1 teaspoon dried rosemary
- Salt and pepper to taste
- Fresh parsley for garnish (optional)

Directions:

1. Heat the olive oil in a large pot over medium heat. Add the onion, carrots, and celery, and sauté until softened, about 5 minutes.
2. Add the garlic to the pot and cook for another minute.
3. Stir in the pearl barley, vegetable broth, diced tomatoes, thyme, and rosemary. Bring the soup to a simmer.
4. Cook for 30-35 minutes, until the barley is tender.
5. Season the soup with salt and pepper to taste.
6. Serve hot, garnished with fresh parsley if desired.

Servings: 6

Nutritional Information (per serving):

Calories: 240 kcal
Total Fat: 3g
Saturated Fat: 0.5g
Trans Fat: 0g
Cholesterol: 0mg
Sodium: 800mg
Total Carbohydrates: 47g
Dietary Fiber: 11g
Sugars: 7g

Protein: 9g

4. Roasted Butternut Squash Soup

Ingredients:

- 1 butternut squash, peeled, seeded, and diced
- 1 onion, diced
- 2 carrots, diced
- 2 cloves garlic, minced
- 4 cups vegetable broth
- 1 teaspoon ground cumin
- 1/2 teaspoon ground cinnamon
- Salt and pepper to taste
- Greek yogurt for serving (optional)

Directions:

1. Set oven temperature to 400°F, or 200°C. After putting the chopped butternut squash on a baking sheet, roast it for 25 to 30 minutes, or until it's soft and has a light brown color.
2. Warm up the olive oil in a big saucepan over medium heat. Add the garlic, onion, and carrots. After around five minutes, sauté until softened.
3. Add the roasted butternut squash to the pot, along with the vegetable broth, cumin, and cinnamon. Bring to a simmer.
4. Cook for 15-20 minutes, allowing the flavors to meld together.
5. Use an immersion blender to puree the soup until smooth. Alternatively, carefully transfer the soup in batches to a blender and blend until smooth.
6. Season the soup with salt and pepper to taste.
7. Serve hot, with a dollop of Greek yogurt if desired.

Servings: 4

Nutritional Information (per serving):

Calories: 180 kcal

Total Fat: 1g

Saturated Fat: 0g

Trans Fat: 0g

Cholesterol: 0mg

Sodium: 780mg

Total Carbohydrates: 43g

Dietary Fiber: 8g

Sugars: 10g

Protein: 4g

5. Hearty Vegetable Quinoa Soup

Ingredients:

- 1 tablespoon olive oil
- 1 onion, diced
- 2 carrots, diced
- 2 celery stalks, diced
- 2 cloves garlic, minced
- 1 cup quinoa, rinsed
- 6 cups vegetable broth
- 1 can (14 oz) diced tomatoes
- 2 cups chopped kale
- 1 teaspoon dried thyme
- 1 teaspoon dried basil
- Salt and pepper to taste
- Fresh parsley for garnish (optional)

Directions:

1. Heat the olive oil in a large pot over medium heat. Add the onion, carrots, and celery, and sauté until softened, about 5 minutes.
2. Add the garlic to the pot and cook for another minute.
3. Stir in the quinoa, vegetable broth, diced tomatoes, kale, thyme, and basil. Bring the soup to a simmer.
4. Cook for 15-20 minutes, until the quinoa is cooked and the vegetables are tender.
5. Season the soup with salt and pepper to taste.
6. Serve hot, garnished with fresh parsley if desired.

Servings: 6

Nutritional Information (per serving):

Calories: 240 kcal

Total Fat: 4g

Saturated Fat: 0.5g

Trans Fat: 0g

Cholesterol: 0mg

Sodium: 850mg

Total Carbohydrates: 45g

Dietary Fiber: 8g

Sugars: 7g

Protein: 9g

4.2 Refreshing Zero Point Salad Creations

1. Summer Citrus Salad

Ingredients:

- 2 cups mixed salad greens (such as lettuce, spinach, or arugula)
- 1 orange, segmented
- 1 grapefruit, segmented
- 1/2 cucumber, sliced
- 1/4 red onion, thinly sliced
- 2 tablespoons fresh mint leaves, chopped
- Juice of 1 lemon
- Salt and pepper to taste

Directions:

1. In a large bowl, combine the mixed salad greens, orange segments, grapefruit segments, cucumber slices, red onion slices, and chopped mint leaves.
2. Squeeze the lemon juice over the salad and toss to combine.
3. Season with salt and pepper to taste.
4. Serve immediately and enjoy!

Servings: 2

Nutritional Information (per serving):

Calories: 70 kcal

Total Fat: 0.5g

Saturated Fat: 0g

Trans Fat: 0g

Cholesterol: 0mg

Sodium: 15mg

Total Carbohydrates: 17g

Dietary Fiber: 4g

Sugars: 10g

Protein: 2g

2. Greek Cucumber Salad

Ingredients:

- 2 large cucumbers, diced
- 1 cup cherry tomatoes, halved
- 1/4 red onion, thinly sliced
- 1/4 cup Kalamata olives, pitted
- Two tablespoons of feta cheese, crumbled
- Two tablespoons freshly cut parsley and one lemon's juice
- 1 tablespoon extra virgin olive oil
- Salt and pepper to taste

Directions:

1. In a large bowl, combine the diced cucumbers, cherry tomatoes, red onion slices, Kalamata olives, crumbled feta cheese, and chopped parsley.
2. Drizzle the lemon juice and olive oil over the salad.
3. Toss to combine.
4. Season with salt and pepper to taste.
5. Serve immediately and enjoy!

Servings: 2

Nutritional Information (per serving):

Calories: 150 kcal

Total Fat: 11g

Saturated Fat: 2.5g

Trans Fat: 0g

Cholesterol: 5mg

Sodium: 270mg

Total Carbohydrates: 13g

Dietary Fiber: 4g

Sugars: 6g

Protein: 4g

3. Watermelon Feta Salad

Ingredients:

- 2 cups cubed watermelon
- 1/2 cucumber, diced
- 1/4 red onion, thinly sliced
- 2 tablespoons crumbled feta cheese
- 2 tablespoons fresh mint leaves, chopped
- Juice of 1 lime
- Salt and pepper to taste

Directions:

1. In a large bowl, combine the cubed watermelon, diced cucumber, red onion slices, crumbled feta cheese, and chopped mint leaves.
2. Squeeze the lime juice over the salad.
3. Toss to combine.
4. Season with salt and pepper to taste.
5. Serve immediately and enjoy!

Servings: 2

Nutritional Information (per serving):

Calories: 90 kcal

Total Fat: 2g

Saturated Fat: 1g

Trans Fat: 0g

Cholesterol: 5mg

Sodium: 120mg

Total Carbohydrates: 18g

Dietary Fiber: 2g

Sugars: 14g

Protein: 2g

4. Asian Cabbage Salad

Ingredients:

- Two cups of shredded purple or green cabbage
- Half a red bell pepper, cut thinly
- 1/2 of a julienned carrot
- Two tsp finely chopped green onions
- two teaspoons of finely chopped cilantro
- One spoonful of seeds from sesame
- 1 tablespoon low-sodium soy sauce
- 1 tablespoon rice vinegar
- 1 teaspoon sesame oil
- 1/2 teaspoon honey
- Salt and pepper to taste

Directions:

1. In a large bowl, combine the shredded cabbage, sliced red bell pepper, julienned carrot, sliced green onions, chopped cilantro, and sesame seeds.
2. In a small bowl, whisk together the soy sauce, rice vinegar, sesame oil, and honey.
3. After adding the dressing to the salad, stir to mix.
4. Season with salt and pepper to taste.
5. Serve immediately and enjoy!

Servings: 2

Nutritional Information (per serving):

Calories: 80 kcal
Total Fat: 4g
Saturated Fat: 0.5g
Trans Fat: 0g
Cholesterol: 0mg
Sodium: 350mg
Total Carbohydrates: 10g
Dietary Fiber: 3g
Sugars: 5g
Protein: 3g

5. Caprese Salad Skewers

Ingredients:

- 1 cup cherry tomatoes
- 1 cup fresh mozzarella balls (bocconcini)
- 1/4 cup fresh basil leaves
- 1 tablespoon balsamic glaze
- Salt and pepper to taste

Directions:

1. Thread a cherry tomato, a mozzarella ball, and a basil leaf onto each skewer.
2. Place the skewers on a dish for serving.
3. Drizzle the balsamic glaze over the skewers.
4. Season with salt and pepper to taste.
5. Serve immediately and enjoy!

Servings: 2 (makes about 6 skewers)

Nutritional Information (per serving, 3 skewers):

Calories: 150 kcal
Total Fat: 10g
Saturated Fat: 6g
Trans Fat: 0g
Cholesterol: 30mg
Sodium: 250mg
Total Carbohydrates: 6g
Dietary Fiber: 1g
Sugars: 3g
Protein: 10g

4.3 Wholesome Broths and Stews for Comfort

1. Classic Chicken Noodle Soup

Ingredients:

- 1 tablespoon olive oil
- 1 onion, diced
- 2 carrots, sliced
- 2 celery stalks, sliced
- 2 cloves garlic, minced
- 6 cups chicken broth
- 2 cups cooked chicken breast, shredded
- 1 cup uncooked egg noodles
- 2 tablespoons fresh parsley, chopped
- Salt and pepper to taste

Directions:

1. Warm up the olive oil in a big saucepan over medium heat. Add the garlic, celery, carrots, and onion. After around five minutes, sauté until softened.
2. Add the chicken broth and heat until it boils.
3. To the saucepan, add the egg noodles and the shredded chicken. Simmer the noodles for 8 to 10 minutes, or until they are soft.
4. Add the parsley that has been chopped and season with salt and pepper to taste.
5. Enjoy it while it's hot!

Servings: 4

Nutritional Information (per serving):

Calories: 250 kcal

Total Fat: 8g

Saturated Fat: 2g

Trans Fat: 0g

Cholesterol: 60mg

Sodium: 780mg

Total Carbohydrates: 18g

Dietary Fiber: 2g

Sugars: 3g

Protein: 24g

2. Hearty Beef and Vegetable Stew

Ingredients:

- 1 tablespoon olive oil
- 1 lb beef stew meat, cubed
- 1 onion, diced
- 2 carrots, sliced
- 2 celery stalks, sliced
- 2 cloves garlic, minced
- 4 cups beef broth
- 2 cups diced potatoes
- 1 cup frozen peas
- 1 teaspoon dried thyme
- Salt and pepper to taste

Directions:

1. Warm up the olive oil in a big saucepan over medium-high heat. After adding the beef stew meat, cook it for about five minutes on both sides.
2. To the saucepan, add the onion, celery, carrots, and garlic. Cook for approximately 5 minutes, or until the veggies start to soften.
3. Add the beef broth and boil for a while. Cook for 1 hour, stirring occasionally.
4. Add the diced potatoes, frozen peas, and dried thyme to the pot. Cook until the potatoes are tender, about 20-25 minutes.
5. To taste, add salt and pepper for seasoning.

6. Enjoy it while it's hot!

Servings: 6

Nutritional Information (per serving):

Calories: 320 kcal

Total Fat: 10g

Saturated Fat: 3g

Trans Fat: 0g

Cholesterol: 70mg

Sodium: 780mg

Total Carbohydrates: 24g

Dietary Fiber: 4g

Sugars: 4g

Protein: 32g

3. Lentil and Vegetable Soup

Ingredients:

- 1 tablespoon olive oil
- 1 onion, diced
- 2 carrots, diced
- 2 celery stalks, diced
- 2 cloves garlic, minced
- 1 cup dried green lentils, rinsed
- 6 cups vegetable broth
- 1 can (14 oz) diced tomatoes
- 2 cups chopped spinach
- 1 teaspoon ground cumin
- Salt and pepper to taste

Directions:

1. In a large pot, heat olive oil over medium heat. Add the onion, carrots, celery, and garlic. Sauté until softened, about 5 minutes.
2. Add the dried green lentils, vegetable broth, diced tomatoes, chopped spinach, and ground cumin to the pot. Bring to a boil, then reduce heat and simmer for 30-35 minutes, or until the lentils are tender.
3. Season with salt and pepper to taste.
4. Serve hot and enjoy!

Servings: 6

Nutritional Information (per serving):

Calories: 230 kcal
Total Fat: 3g
Saturated Fat: 0g
Trans Fat: 0g
Cholesterol: 0mg
Sodium: 780mg
Total Carbohydrates: 40g
Dietary Fiber: 15g
Sugars: 5g
Protein: 13g

4. Creamy Potato Leek Soup

Ingredients:

- 2 tablespoons unsalted butter
- 2 leeks, white and light green parts only, sliced
- 4 cups diced potatoes
- 4 cups chicken or vegetable broth
- 1 cup milk or cream

- Salt and pepper to taste
- Chopped chives for garnish (optional)

Directions:

1. Melt the butter in a big saucepan over a medium heat. Slicing the leeks should take around 5 minutes to soften.
2. Pour the liquid and cubed potatoes into the pot. After bringing to a boil, lower the heat and simmer the potatoes for 15 to 20 minutes, or until they are soft.
3. Puree the soup with an immersion blender until it's smooth. Alternatively, put the soup to a blender and process until smooth, working in batches.
4. Add the cream or milk and stir, then fully heat.
5. To taste, add salt and pepper for seasoning.
6. Serve hot, garnished with chopped chives if desired.

Servings: 4

Nutritional Information (per serving):

Calories: 280 kcal
Total Fat: 8g
Saturated Fat: 5g
Trans Fat: 0g
Cholesterol: 25mg
Sodium: 700mg
Total Carbohydrates: 45g
Dietary Fiber: 6g
Sugars: 6g
Protein: 8g

5. Moroccan Chickpea Stew

Ingredients:

- 1 tablespoon olive oil

- 1 onion, diced
- 2 carrots, diced
- 2 celery stalks, diced
- 2 cloves garlic, minced
- 1 teaspoon ground cumin
- 1 teaspoon ground coriander
- 1/2 teaspoon ground cinnamon
- 1/4 teaspoon ground turmeric
- 1 can (15 oz) chickpeas, drained and rinsed
- 1 can (14 oz) diced tomatoes
- 4 cups vegetable broth
- 1/4 cup chopped fresh cilantro
- Salt and pepper to taste

Directions:

1. In a large pot, heat olive oil over medium heat. Add the onion, carrots, celery, and garlic. Sauté until softened, about 5 minutes.
2. Add the ground cumin, ground coriander, ground cinnamon, and ground turmeric to the pot. Cook for 1 minute, until fragrant.
3. Stir in the chickpeas, diced tomatoes, and vegetable broth. Bring to a boil, then reduce heat and simmer for 20-25 minutes.
4. Season with salt and pepper to taste.
5. Serve hot, garnished with chopped fresh cilantro.

Servings: 4

Nutritional Information (per serving):

Calories: 230 kcal
Total Fat: 4g
Saturated Fat: 0.5g
Trans Fat: 0g
Cholesterol: 0mg
Sodium: 680mg

Total Carbohydrates: 40g
Dietary Fiber: 12g
Sugars: 9g
Protein: 9g

Adjust ingredients and servings as needed to fit your personal dietary preferences and requirements. Enjoy these wholesome broths and stews for comforting meals!

Chapter 5: Delicious Main Courses

5.1 Zesty Zero Point Chicken Dishes

Lemon Herb Grilled Chicken:

Ingredients:

- 4 boneless, skinless chicken breasts
- Zest and juice of 1 lemon
- 2 cloves garlic, minced
- 2 tablespoons chopped fresh herbs (such as rosemary, thyme, or parsley)
- Salt and pepper to taste

Directions:

1. In a small bowl, whisk together the lemon zest, lemon juice, minced garlic, chopped herbs, salt, and pepper to create a marinade.
2. After putting the chicken breasts in a shallow dish, cover them completely with the marinade. For a minimum of half an hour and a maximum of four hours, cover and chill.
3. Set the grill's temperature to medium-high. Take the chicken out of the marinade and throw away any extra marinade.
4. Grill chicken for 6-8 minutes per side, or until cooked through and juices run clear.
5. Serve hot and enjoy the zesty flavor of lemon herb grilled chicken.

Spicy Buffalo Chicken Lettuce Wraps:

Ingredients:

- 1 pound of cooked, shredded, skinless, boneless chicken breasts
- 1/2 cup hot sauce (choose a brand with zero points)
- 1 tablespoon unsalted butter
- Iceberg lettuce leaves, for wrapping
- Optional toppings: shredded carrots, diced celery, ranch or blue cheese dressing

Directions:
1. In a skillet over medium heat, combine the hot sauce and unsalted butter. Cook until the butter is melted and the sauce is heated through.
2. Add the shredded chicken to the skillet and toss until evenly coated with the buffalo sauce.
3. Spoon the buffalo chicken mixture onto iceberg lettuce leaves, dividing evenly among them.
4. Top with optional toppings such as shredded carrots, diced celery, and a drizzle of ranch or blue cheese dressing.
5. Roll up the lettuce leaves to create wraps and serve immediately for a zesty and satisfying meal.

Tangy Balsamic Chicken Skewers:

Ingredients:
- 1 lb boneless, skinless chicken breasts, cut into cubes
- 1/4 cup balsamic vinegar
- 2 tablespoons Dijon mustard
- 1 tablespoon honey
- 2 cloves garlic, minced
- Salt and pepper to taste

Directions:
1. In a bowl, whisk together the balsamic vinegar, Dijon mustard, honey, minced garlic, salt, and pepper to create a marinade.
2. After adding the chicken cubes to the marinade, toss to coat them completely. For at least 30 minutes and up to two hours, cover and chill.
3. Turn the heat up to medium-high on the grill or grill pan. After marinating, thread the chicken cubes onto skewers.
4. Grill the chicken skewers for 5-6 minutes per side, or until cooked through and slightly charred.
5. Serve hot, garnished with fresh herbs if desired, and enjoy the tangy flavor of balsamic chicken skewers.

Garlic Lime Chicken Stir-Fry:

Ingredients:
- 1 lb boneless, skinless chicken breasts, thinly sliced
- Juice of 2 limes
- Zest of 1 lime
- 2 cloves garlic, minced
- 1 tablespoon low-sodium soy sauce
- 1 teaspoon honey
- 1 tablespoon olive oil
- Assorted vegetables (such as bell peppers, snap peas, and broccoli)

Directions:
1. In a bowl, combine the lime juice, lime zest, minced garlic, soy sauce, and honey to create a marinade.
2. Add the sliced chicken to the marinade and toss until well coated. Give it a minimum of fifteen minutes to marinate.
3. In a large skillet or wok, heat the olive oil over medium-high heat. Add the marinated chicken and cook until browned and cooked through, about 5-6 minutes.
4. Add assorted vegetables to the skillet and stir-fry until crisp-tender, about 3-4 minutes.
5. Serve hot and enjoy the vibrant flavors of garlic lime chicken stir-fry.

5.2 Flavorful Fish and Seafood Entrees

1. Lemon Garlic Grilled Salmon

Ingredients:

- 2 salmon filets (6 oz each)
- 2 cloves garlic, minced
- Zest and juice of 1 lemon
- 2 tablespoons olive oil
- Salt and pepper to taste
- Fresh parsley for garnish

Directions:

1. In a small bowl, mix together the minced garlic, lemon zest, lemon juice, olive oil, salt, and pepper.
2. Pour the marinade over the salmon fillets and place them in a shallow dish. Give it a half hour to marinate.
3. Set the grill's temperature to medium-high.
4. Take the salmon out of the marinade and throw away any extra marinade.
5. When the salmon fillets are cooked through and can be easily flaked with a fork, place them on the grill and cook for 4–5 minutes on each side.
6. Serve hot, garnished with fresh parsley.

Servings: 2

Nutritional Information (per serving):

Calories: 350 kcal

Total Fat: 21g

Saturated Fat: 3g

Trans Fat: 0g

Cholesterol: 90mg

Sodium: 70mg

Total Carbohydrates: 2g

Dietary Fiber: 0g

Sugars: 0g

Protein: 35g

2. Shrimp Scampi

Ingredients:

- 1 lb large shrimp, peeled and deveined
- 4 cloves garlic, minced
- 1/4 cup white wine
- 2 tablespoons lemon juice
- 2 tablespoons unsalted butter
- 2 tablespoons olive oil
- Salt and pepper to taste
- Fresh parsley for garnish
- Crusty bread or cooked spaghetti to serve (optional)

Directions:

1. Heat the olive oil in a big skillet over medium heat. Add the minced garlic and sauté until fragrant, about 1 minute.
2. When the shrimp are pink and opaque, add them to the skillet and cook for two to three minutes on each side.
3. After taking the shrimp out of the pan, set it aside.
4. Using white wine, deglaze the skillet, being sure to scrape away any browned pieces from the pan's bottom.
5. Stir in the lemon juice and unsalted butter until the butter is melted and the sauce is combined.
6. Put the shrimp back in the skillet and toss them around to cover with sauce.
7. Season with salt and pepper to taste.

8. Garnish with fresh parsley and serve hot, with cooked pasta or crusty bread if desired.

Servings: 4

Nutritional Information (per serving, without pasta or bread):

Calories: 190 kcal

Total Fat: 12g

Saturated Fat: 4g

Trans Fat: 0g

Cholesterol: 175mg

Sodium: 230mg

Total Carbohydrates: 3g

Dietary Fiber: 0g

Sugars: 0g

Protein: 18g

3. Baked Lemon Garlic Butter Cod

Ingredients:

- 2 cod filets (6 oz each)
- 2 cloves garlic, minced
- Zest and juice of 1 lemon
- 2 tablespoons unsalted butter, melted
- Salt and pepper to taste
- Fresh parsley for garnish

Directions:

1. Set oven temperature to 400°F, or 200°C. Grease a baking dish very lightly.
2. In a small bowl, mix together the minced garlic, lemon zest, lemon juice, melted butter, salt, and pepper.
3. Place the cod filets in the prepared baking dish and pour the lemon garlic butter mixture over them.

4. Bake for 12 to 15 minutes, or until a fork can easily pierce the fish, in a preheated oven.

5. Garnish with fresh parsley and serve hot.

Servings: 2

Nutritional Information (per serving):

Calories: 230 kcal

Total Fat: 10g

Saturated Fat: 6g

Trans Fat: 0g

Cholesterol: 80mg

Sodium: 220mg

Total Carbohydrates: 2g

Dietary Fiber: 0g

Sugars: 0g

Protein: 34g

4. Spicy Cajun Grilled Shrimp

Ingredients:

- 1 lb large shrimp, peeled and deveined
- 2 tablespoons olive oil
- 2 teaspoons Cajun seasoning
- 1 teaspoon paprika
- 1/2 teaspoon garlic powder
- 1/2 teaspoon onion powder
- 1/4 teaspoon cayenne pepper (adjust to taste)
- Salt and pepper to taste
- Lemon wedges for serving

Directions:

1. In a large bowl, toss the shrimp with olive oil, Cajun seasoning, paprika, garlic powder, onion powder, cayenne pepper, salt, and pepper until evenly coated.
2. Preheat the grill to medium-high heat.
3. If preferred, thread the shrimp onto skewers.
4. Grill until the shrimp are opaque and pink, about two to three minutes per side.
5. Take off of the grill and serve hot with slices of lemon.

Servings: 4

Nutritional Information (per serving):

Calories: 160 kcal

Total Fat: 8g

Saturated Fat: 1g

Trans Fat: 0g

Cholesterol: 160mg

Sodium: 360mg

Total Carbohydrates: 2g

Dietary Fiber: 0g

Sugars: 0g

Protein: 20g

5. Garlic Butter Scallops

Ingredients:

- 1 lb scallops
- 2 tablespoons unsalted butter
- 2 cloves garlic, minced
- Salt and pepper to taste
- Fresh parsley for garnish
- Lemon wedges for serving

Directions:

1. Pat the scallops dry with paper towels and season with salt and pepper.
2. In a large skillet, melt the unsalted butter over medium-high heat. Add the minced garlic and cook for 1 minute, until fragrant.
3. Add the scallops to the skillet in a single layer, making sure not to overcrowd the pan. Cook for 2-3 minutes per side, until golden brown and cooked through.
4. Remove the scallops from the skillet and garnish with fresh parsley.
5. Serve hot with lemon wedges.

Servings: 4

Nutritional Information (per serving):

Calories: 150 kcal
Total Fat: 6g
Saturated Fat: 3g
Trans Fat: 0g
Cholesterol: 45mg
Sodium: 350mg
Total Carbohydrates: 4g
Dietary Fiber: 0g
Sugars: 0g
Protein: 20g

5.3 Savory Vegetarian and Vegan Options

1. Vegetarian Chickpea Curry

Ingredients:

- 2 tablespoons olive oil
- 1 onion, diced
- 2 cloves garlic, minced
- 1 tablespoon grated ginger
- 1 tablespoon curry powder
- 1 teaspoon ground cumin
- 1 teaspoon ground turmeric
- 1 can (15 oz) chickpeas, drained and rinsed
- 1 can (14 oz) diced tomatoes
- 1 can (13.5 oz) coconut milk
- Salt and pepper to taste
- Fresh cilantro for garnish
- Cooked rice or naan for serving

Directions:

1. In a big skillet over medium heat, warm up the olive oil. Add the grated ginger, minced garlic, and chopped onion. Sauté for about 5 minutes, or until onions are tender and transparent.
2. Add the ground turmeric, cumin, and curry powder and stir. Simmer for a further one to two minutes, or until aromatic.
3. To the pan, add the chopped tomatoes, chickpeas, and coconut milk. Bring to a boil and cook, stirring periodically, for 15 to 20 minutes.
4. To taste, add salt and pepper for seasoning.
5. Serve hot over cooked rice or with naan, garnished with fresh cilantro.

Servings: 4

Nutritional Information (per serving, without rice or naan):

Calories: 320 kcal

Total Fat: 20g

Saturated Fat: 12g

Trans Fat: 0g

Cholesterol: 0mg

Sodium: 340mg

Total Carbohydrates: 30g

Dietary Fiber: 9g

Sugars: 7g

Protein: 8g

2. Vegan Lentil Shepherd's Pie

Ingredients:

- 2 cups cooked lentils
- 1 onion, diced
- 2 carrots, diced
- 2 celery stalks, diced
- 2 cloves garlic, minced
- 1 cup frozen peas
- 1 cup vegetable broth
- 2 tablespoons tomato paste
- 1 teaspoon dried thyme
- Mashed potatoes (prepared separately)
- Salt and pepper to taste

Directions:

1. Turn the oven on to 375°F, or 190°C. Grease a baking dish very lightly.
2. In a large skillet, sauté diced onion, carrots, celery, and minced garlic until softened, about 5 minutes.

3. Add cooked lentils, frozen peas, vegetable broth, tomato paste, and dried thyme to the skillet. Cook for an additional 5-7 minutes, until heated through and the mixture thickens slightly.
4. Season with salt and pepper to taste.
5. Transfer the lentil mixture to the prepared baking dish. Top with mashed potatoes, spreading them evenly over the lentil mixture.
6. Bake in the preheated oven for 20-25 minutes, or until the mashed potatoes are lightly golden on top.
7. Serve hot.

Servings: 4

Nutritional Information (per serving):

Calories: 280 kcal
Total Fat: 1g
Saturated Fat: 0g
Trans Fat: 0g
Cholesterol: 0mg
Sodium: 400mg
Total Carbohydrates: 54g
Dietary Fiber: 16g
Sugars: 10g
Protein: 17g

3. Vegan Mushroom Stroganoff

Ingredients:

- 8 oz pasta of choice (such as fettuccine or penne)
- 2 tablespoons olive oil
- 1 onion, diced
- 2 cloves garlic, minced
- 8 oz mushrooms, sliced

- One tablespoon all-purpose flour
- One cup vegetable broth
- 1 cup unsweetened almond milk
- 2 tablespoons nutritional yeast
- 1 tablespoon soy sauce
- Salt and pepper to taste
- Fresh parsley for garnish

Directions:

1. Follow the directions on the package to cook the pasta. After draining, set away.
2. Heat the olive oil in a big skillet over medium heat. Add chopped onion and minced garlic, and cook for about 5 minutes, or until softened.
3. Sliced mushrooms should be added to the skillet and cooked for five to seven minutes, or until they release moisture and become soft.
4. After dusting the mushrooms with all-purpose flour, toss to coat them evenly. Simmer for one or two more minutes.
5. Slowly pour in vegetable broth and unsweetened almond milk, stirring constantly until the mixture thickens, about 5 minutes.
6. Stir in nutritional yeast and soy sauce. To taste, add salt and pepper for seasoning.
7. When the pasta is done, add it to the skillet and toss to cover with sauce.
8. Garnish with fresh parsley and serve hot.

Servings: 4

Nutritional Information (per serving):

Calories: 350 kcal

Total Fat: 10g

Saturated Fat: 1g

Trans Fat: 0g

Cholesterol: 0mg

Sodium: 300mg

Total Carbohydrates: 55g

Dietary Fiber: 5g

Sugars: 3g

Protein: 12g

4. Vegetarian Eggplant Parmesan

Ingredients:

- 2 large eggplants, sliced into rounds
- 2 cups marinara sauce
- 1 cup breadcrumbs
- 1/2 cup grated Parmesan cheese (or nutritional yeast for vegan option)
- 2 tablespoons olive oil
- 2 cloves garlic, minced
- Salt and pepper to taste
- For garnish, use fresh basil leaves.

Directions:

1. Set oven temperature to 400°F, or 200°C. Grease a baking sheet very lightly.
2. Arrange the circles of eggplant on the baking sheet. Drizzle the eggplant slices with olive oil and season with minced garlic. Add pepper and salt for seasoning.
3. Bake the eggplant for 20 to 25 minutes in a preheated oven, or until it is soft and browned.
4. From the oven, remove the eggplant. Lower the oven's setting to 175°C/350°F.
5. In a separate bowl, mix together breadcrumbs and grated Parmesan cheese.
6. In a baking dish, layer marinara sauce, baked eggplant slices, and breadcrumb mixture. Repeat layers until all ingredients are used, ending with a layer of breadcrumbs on top.
7. Bake for 25 to 30 minutes, or until bubbling and brown on top.
8. Garnish with fresh basil leaves and serve hot.

Servings: 4

Nutritional Information (per serving):

Calories: 320 kcal

Total Fat: 10g

Saturated Fat: 2g

Trans Fat: 0g

Cholesterol: 5mg

Sodium: 700mg

Total Carbohydrates: 50g

Dietary Fiber: 12g

Sugars: 12g

Protein: 10g

5. Vegan Black Bean Tacos

Ingredients:

- 8 small corn tortillas
- 2 cups cooked black beans
- 1 avocado, sliced
- 1 cup shredded lettuce
- 1/2 cup diced tomatoes
- 1/4 cup diced red onion
- 1/4 cup chopped fresh cilantro
- Juice of 1 lime
- Salt and pepper to taste
- Hot sauce or salsa for serving (optional)

Directions:

1. Warm the corn tortillas in a dry skillet over medium heat until soft and pliable.
2. Fill each tortilla with cooked black beans, avocado slices, shredded lettuce, diced tomatoes, diced red onion, and chopped fresh cilantro.
3. Squeeze lime juice over the taco fillings and season with salt and pepper to taste.

4. Serve hot with hot sauce or salsa on the side, if desired.

Servings: 4 (2 tacos per serving)

Nutritional Information (per serving, 2 tacos):

Calories: 350 kcal

Total Fat: 12g

Saturated Fat: 2g

Trans Fat: 0g

Cholesterol: 0mg

Sodium: 250mg

Total Carbohydrates: 52g

Dietary Fiber: 16g

Sugars: 3g

Protein: 12g

Chapter 6: Mouthwatering Side Dishes

6.1 Vibrant Vegetable Sides to Complement Any Meal

1. Roasted Garlic Parmesan Green Beans

Ingredients:

- 1 lb green beans, trimmed
- 2 tablespoons olive oil
- 2 cloves garlic, minced
- 1/4 cup of Parmesan cheese, grated
- To taste, add salt and pepper.

Directions:

1. Set the oven temperature to 425°F (220°C).
2. In a large bowl, toss the green beans with olive oil, minced garlic, grated Parmesan cheese, salt, and pepper until evenly coated.
3. Spread the green beans in a single layer on a baking sheet.
4. Roast in the preheated oven for 15-20 minutes, or until the green beans are tender and slightly browned.
5. Serve hot.

Servings: 4

Nutritional Information (per serving):

Calories: 120 kcal
Total Fat: 7g
Saturated Fat: 2g
Trans Fat: 0g
Cholesterol: 5mg

Sodium: 140mg

Total Carbohydrates: 10g

Dietary Fiber: 4g

Sugars: 3g

Protein: 4g

2. Honey Glazed Carrots

Ingredients:

- 1 lb carrots, peeled and sliced
- 2 tablespoons butter
- 2 tablespoons honey
- Salt and pepper to taste
- For garnish, use fresh parsley (optional).

Directions:

1. Heat a large pan over medium heat to melt the butter.
2. Add the sliced carrots to the skillet and cook for 3-4 minutes, stirring occasionally.
3. Drizzle the honey over the carrots and continue cooking for another 5-6 minutes, or until the carrots are tender and caramelized.
4. Season with salt and pepper to taste.
5. If desired, garnish with fresh parsley.
6. Warm up the food.

Servings: 4

Nutritional Information (per serving):

Calories: 120 kcal

Total Fat: 5g

Saturated Fat: 3g

Trans Fat: 0g

Cholesterol: 15mg

Sodium: 130mg

Total Carbohydrates: 20g

Dietary Fiber: 3g

Sugars: 14g

Protein: 1g

3. Balsamic Glazed Brussels Sprouts

Ingredients:

- One pound of trimmed and halved Brussels sprouts
- Two tsp olive oil
- 2 tablespoons balsamic vinegar
- 1 tablespoon honey
- Salt and pepper to taste

Directions:

1. Set oven temperature to 400°F, or 200°C.
2. In a large bowl, toss the Brussels sprouts with olive oil, balsamic vinegar, honey, salt, and pepper until evenly coated.
3. Spread the Brussels sprouts in a single layer on a baking sheet.
4. Roast in the preheated oven for 20-25 minutes, or until the Brussels sprouts are tender and caramelized.
5. Serve hot.

Servings: 4

Nutritional Information (per serving):

Calories: 110 kcal

Total Fat: 5g

Saturated Fat: 1g

Trans Fat: 0g

Cholesterol: 0mg

Sodium: 25mg

Total Carbohydrates: 15g

Dietary Fiber: 4g

Sugars: 7g

Protein: 4g

4. Lemon Garlic Roasted Asparagus

Ingredients:

- 1 lb asparagus, trimmed
- 2 tablespoons olive oil
- 2 cloves garlic, minced
- Zest and juice of 1 lemon
- Salt and pepper to taste

Directions:

1. Preheat the oven to 425°F (220°C).
2. In a large bowl, toss the asparagus with olive oil, minced garlic, lemon zest, lemon juice, salt, and pepper until evenly coated.
3. Spread the asparagus in a single layer on a baking sheet.
4. Roast in the preheated oven for 10-12 minutes, or until the asparagus is tender and slightly browned.
5. Serve hot.

Servings: 4

Nutritional Information (per serving):

Calories: 70 kcal

Total Fat: 5g

Saturated Fat: 1g

Trans Fat: 0g

Cholesterol: 0mg

Sodium: 5mg

Total Carbohydrates: 6g
Dietary Fiber: 2g
Sugars: 2g
Protein: 2g

6.2 Delectable Grain and Legume-Based Sides

1. Quinoa and Black Bean Salad

Ingredients:

- 1 cup quinoa, rinsed
- two cups of veggie broth or water
- One can (15 oz) of rinsed and drained black beans
- One sliced bell pepper, one cup cherry tomatoes, one halved, and one-fourth cup finely chopped red onion
- 1/4 cup fresh cilantro, chopped
- Juice of 1 lime
- 2 tablespoons olive oil
- Salt and pepper to taste

Directions:

1. Bring water or vegetable broth to a boil in a medium-sized pot. After adding the quinoa, lower the heat to a simmer, cover, and let the quinoa cook for 15 to 20 minutes, or until the liquid has been absorbed. Turn off the heat and let it to cool.
2. In a large bowl, combine cooked quinoa, black beans, diced bell pepper, cherry tomatoes, red onion, and fresh cilantro.
3. In a small bowl, whisk together lime juice, olive oil, salt, and pepper. Pour over the quinoa mixture and toss until well combined.
4. Serve chilled or at room temperature.

Servings: 4

Nutritional Information (per serving):

Calories: 290 kcal

Total Fat: 8g

Saturated Fat: 1g

Trans Fat: 0g

Cholesterol: 0mg

Sodium: 300mg

Total Carbohydrates: 45g

Dietary Fiber: 10g

Sugars: 3g

Protein: 11g

2. Mediterranean Chickpea Salad

Ingredients:

- Two cans (15 oz each) of rinsed and drained chickpeas
- one chopped cucumber
- 1 cup cherry tomatoes, halved
- 1/4 cup red onion, finely chopped
- 1/4 cup Kalamata olives, pitted and sliced
- 1/4 cup fresh parsley, chopped
- 2 tablespoons lemon juice
- 2 tablespoons extra virgin olive oil
- 1 teaspoon dried oregano
- Salt and pepper to taste

Directions:

1. In a large bowl, combine chickpeas, diced cucumber, cherry tomatoes, red onion, Kalamata olives, and fresh parsley.
2. In a small bowl, whisk together lemon juice, extra virgin olive oil, dried oregano, salt, and pepper. Pour over the chickpea mixture and toss until well combined.
3. Serve chilled or at room temperature.

Servings: 4

Nutritional Information (per serving):

Calories: 280 kcal

Total Fat: 11g

Saturated Fat: 1g

Trans Fat: 0g

Cholesterol: 0mg

Sodium: 360mg

Total Carbohydrates: 37g

Dietary Fiber: 10g

Sugars: 6g

Protein: 11g

3. Brown Rice Pilaf with Lentils

Ingredients:

- 1 cup brown rice
- 2 cups vegetable broth
- 1/2 cup dried green lentils
- 1 onion, diced
- 2 cloves garlic, minced
- 2 carrots, diced
- 2 stalks celery, diced
- 1 tablespoon olive oil
- Salt and pepper to taste
- For garnish, use fresh parsley (optional).

Directions:

1. Olive oil should be heated over medium heat in a big saucepan. Add diced onion and minced garlic, and sauté until softened, about 5 minutes.
2. Add diced carrots and celery to the saucepan and cook for another 3-4 minutes.

3. Stir in brown rice, vegetable broth, and dried green lentils. Bring to a boil, then reduce heat to low, cover, and simmer for 40-45 minutes, or until rice and lentils are cooked and liquid is absorbed.
4. To taste, add salt and pepper for seasoning. Using a fork, fluff.
5. If desired, garnish with fresh parsley.
6. Warm up the food.

Servings: 4

Nutritional Information (per serving):

Calories: 280 kcal
Total Fat: 3.5g
Saturated Fat: 0.5g
Trans Fat: 0g
Cholesterol: 0mg
Sodium: 380mg
Total Carbohydrates: 52g
Dietary Fiber: 9g
Sugars: 4g
Protein: 11g

4. Couscous with Roasted Vegetables

Ingredients:

- 1 cup couscous
- 1 1/4 cups vegetable broth
- 1 bell pepper, diced
- 1 zucchini, diced
- 1 yellow squash, diced
- 1 red onion, sliced
- 2 tablespoons olive oil

- 1 teaspoon ground cumin
- 1 teaspoon paprika
- Salt and pepper to taste
- Fresh parsley for garnish (optional)

Directions:

1. Set oven temperature to 400°F, or 200°C.
2. In a large bowl, toss diced bell pepper, zucchini, yellow squash, and sliced red onion with olive oil, ground cumin, paprika, salt, and pepper until evenly coated.
3. Spread the vegetables in a single layer on a baking sheet.
4. Roast in the preheated oven for 20-25 minutes, or until the vegetables are tender and lightly browned.
5. Meanwhile, in a medium saucepan, bring vegetable broth to a boil. Stir in couscous, cover, and remove from heat. Let it sit for 5 minutes, then fluff with a fork.
6. Transfer the cooked couscous to a serving dish and top with roasted vegetables.
7. If desired, garnish with fresh parsley.
8. Serve hot or at room temperature.

Servings: 4

Nutritional Information (per serving):

Calories: 250 kcal
Total Fat: 7g
Saturated Fat: 1g
Trans Fat: 0g
Cholesterol: 0mg
Sodium: 490mg
Total Carbohydrates: 42g
Dietary Fiber: 5g
Sugars: 5g
Protein: 7g

5. Wild Rice and Mushroom Pilaf

Ingredients:

- 1 cup wild rice
- 2 1/2 cups vegetable broth
- 8 oz mushrooms, sliced
- 1 onion, diced
- 2 cloves garlic, minced
- 2 tablespoons olive oil
- 2 tablespoons fresh thyme leaves
- Salt and pepper to taste

Directions:

1. In a medium saucepan, heat olive oil over medium heat. Add diced onion and minced garlic, and sauté until softened, about 5 minutes.
2. Add sliced mushrooms to the saucepan and cook until they release their moisture and become tender, about 5-7 minutes.
3. Stir in wild rice and fresh thyme leaves. Cook for another 2-3 minutes.
4. Pour vegetable broth into the saucepan and bring to a boil. Reduce heat to low, cover, and simmer for 40-45 minutes, or until rice is tender and liquid is absorbed.
5. Season with salt and pepper to taste.
6. Serve hot.

Servings: 4

Nutritional Information (per serving):

Calories: 220 kcal

Total Fat: 6g

Saturated Fat: 1g

Trans Fat: 0g

Cholesterol: 0mg

Sodium: 480mg

Total Carbohydrates: 35g

Dietary Fiber: 5g

Sugars: 4g

Protein: 7g

6.3 Creative Ways to Incorporate Zero Point Ingredients

1. Veggie-Based "Noodle" Dishes:
Replace traditional pasta with vegetable noodles made from zucchini, carrots, or butternut squash. Make long, thin strands using a vegetable peeler or spiralizer. These veggie noodles can be enjoyed in stir-fries, salads, or topped with marinara sauce for a low-calorie, zero point alternative to pasta.

2. Salad Wraps:
Instead of using tortillas or bread, use large lettuce leaves such as romaine or butterhead lettuce as wraps for your favorite fillings. Fill the lettuce wraps with lean proteins like grilled chicken or shrimp, along with zero point ingredients such as diced tomatoes, cucumbers, bell peppers, and avocado. Drizzle with a low-calorie dressing or salsa for added flavor.

3. Cauliflower Rice Stir-Fry:
Replace traditional rice with cauliflower rice for a low-carb, zero point alternative. Simply pulse cauliflower florets in a food processor until they resemble rice grains, then sauté in a skillet with garlic, onions, and your choice of vegetables. Add in cooked lean protein such as tofu, chicken, or shrimp, and season with soy sauce or your favorite stir-fry sauce for a flavorful and nutritious meal.

4. Greek Yogurt-Based Dips and Dressings:
Greek yogurt is a versatile ingredient that can be used to create creamy dips and dressings without adding extra points. Mix plain non-fat Greek yogurt with herbs, spices, and citrus juice to make a flavorful dip for fresh vegetables or baked chips. You can also use Greek yogurt as a base for salad dressings by adding vinegar, olive oil, mustard, and seasonings.

5. Fruit-Based Desserts:
Enjoy sweet treats without the guilt by incorporating zero point fruits into your desserts. Make a refreshing fruit salad with a variety of colorful fruits such as berries, melons, and citrus fruits. You can also blend frozen bananas with other fruits to create creamy, dairy-free "nice cream" or freeze grapes for a satisfying frozen snack.

6. Eggplant-Based Pizza Crust:
For a gluten-free and low-calorie pizza crust alternative, use slices of roasted eggplant as the base. Simply slice eggplant lengthwise, brush with olive oil, and bake until tender. Top with marinara sauce, vegetables, and low-fat cheese for a satisfying and nutritious pizza option.

7. Cucumber Sushi Rolls:
Replace traditional sushi rice with thinly sliced cucumber for a light and refreshing sushi alternative. Fill the cucumber slices with your favorite sushi ingredients such as avocado, cucumber, carrots, and cooked shrimp or crab. Roll tightly and slice into bite-sized pieces for a zero point snack or appetizer.

These are just a few creative ways to incorporate zero point ingredients into your meals and snacks. By experimenting with different flavors and textures, you can create delicious and satisfying dishes that fit into your healthy eating plan.

Chapter 7: Guilt-Free Snacks and Appetizers

7.1 Crispy Baked Snack Ideas for Any Occasion

1. Baked Sweet Potato Chips

Ingredients:

- 2 medium sweet potatoes, thinly sliced
- 2 tablespoons olive oil
- Salt and pepper to taste

Directions:

1. Before proceeding, preheat the oven to 375°F (190°C) and place parchment paper on a baking pan.
2. Toss the sweet potato slices in a big basin with salt, pepper, and olive oil until well covered.
3. Place the sweet potato slices in a single layer on the baking sheet that has been preheated.
4. The chips should be baked for 15 to 20 minutes in a preheated oven, turning them over halfway through, until they are crispy and golden brown.
5. Take it out of the oven and let it to cool down a little before serving.

Servings: 4

Nutritional Information (per serving):

Calories: 120 kcal

Total Fat: 7g

Saturated Fat: 1g

Trans Fat: 0g

Cholesterol: 0mg

Sodium: 120mg

Total Carbohydrates: 14g

Dietary Fiber: 2g

Sugars: 4g

Protein: 1g

2. Baked Parmesan Zucchini Fries

Ingredients:

- Cut two medium zucchini into fries.
- 1/2 cup grated Parmesan cheese
- 1/4 cup breadcrumbs
- 1 teaspoon garlic powder
- 1 teaspoon dried oregano
- Salt and pepper to taste
- 1 egg, beaten

Directions:

1. Preheat the oven to 425°F (220°C) and line a baking sheet with parchment paper.
2. In a shallow dish, mix together grated Parmesan cheese, breadcrumbs, garlic powder, dried oregano, salt, and pepper.
3. Dip each zucchini fry into the beaten egg, then coat in the Parmesan breadcrumb mixture.
4. Place the coated zucchini fries on the prepared baking sheet in a single layer.
5. Bake in the preheated oven for 20-25 minutes, flipping halfway through, until the fries are crispy and golden brown.
6. Remove from the oven and let cool slightly before serving.

Servings: 4

Nutritional Information (per serving):

Calories: 110 kcal

Total Fat: 5g

Saturated Fat: 2g

Trans Fat: 0g

Cholesterol: 45mg

Sodium: 240mg

Total Carbohydrates: 10g

Dietary Fiber: 2g

Sugars: 3g

Protein: 7g

3. Crispy Baked Chickpeas

Ingredients:

- 1 can (15 oz) chickpeas, drained and rinsed
- 1 tablespoon olive oil
- 1 teaspoon smoked paprika
- 1/2 teaspoon garlic powder
- 1/2 teaspoon cumin
- Salt and pepper to taste

Directions:

1. Adjust the oven temperature to 400°F (200°C) and place parchment paper on a baking pan.
2. Using a paper towel, pat dry the chickpeas and remove any loose skins.
3. Toss the chickpeas in a bowl with olive oil, cumin, garlic powder, smoked paprika, salt, and pepper until well covered.
4. Arrange the seasoned chickpeas on the prepared baking sheet in a single layer.
5. Bake in the preheated oven for 30-35 minutes, shaking the pan halfway through, until the chickpeas are crispy and golden brown.
6. Remove from the oven and let cool slightly before serving.

Servings: 4

Nutritional Information (per serving):

Calories: 120 kcal

Total Fat: 4g

Saturated Fat: 0.5g

Trans Fat: 0g

Cholesterol: 0mg

Sodium: 180mg

Total Carbohydrates: 17g

Dietary Fiber: 5g

Sugars: 0g

Protein: 5g

4. Baked Kale Chips

Ingredients:

- 1 bunch kale, stems removed and torn into bite-sized pieces
- 1 tablespoon olive oil
- Salt and pepper to taste

Directions:

1. Adjust the oven temperature to 350°F (175°C) and place parchment paper on a baking pan.
2. In a large bowl, toss the kale pieces with olive oil, salt, and pepper until evenly coated.
3. Spread the kale in a single layer on the prepared baking sheet.
4. Bake in the preheated oven for 10-15 minutes, checking frequently, until the kale is crispy but not burnt.
5. Remove from the oven and let cool slightly before serving.

Servings: 4

Nutritional Information (per serving):

Calories: 50 kcal

Total Fat: 3g

Saturated Fat: 0g

Trans Fat: 0g

Cholesterol: 0mg

Sodium: 60mg

Total Carbohydrates: 6g

Dietary Fiber: 1g

Sugars: 0g

Protein: 2g

5. Oven-Baked Mozzarella Sticks

Ingredients:

- 8 sticks part-skim mozzarella cheese, cut in half
- half a cup of breadcrumbs made of whole wheat
- 1/4 cup grated Parmesan cheese
- 1 teaspoon Italian seasoning
- 1/2 teaspoon garlic powder
- 1/4 cup all-purpose flour
- 2 eggs, beaten

Directions:

1. Preheat the oven to 400°F (200°C) and line a baking sheet with parchment paper.
2. In a shallow dish, mix together whole wheat breadcrumbs, grated Parmesan cheese, Italian seasoning, and garlic powder.
3. Dredge each mozzarella stick in all-purpose flour, then dip into beaten eggs, and finally coat with breadcrumb mixture, pressing gently to adhere.
4. Arrange the coated mozzarella sticks onto the baking sheet that has been ready.

5. Bake in the preheated oven for 8-10 minutes, or until the cheese is melted and the coating is crispy and golden brown.
6. Remove from the oven and let cool slightly before serving with marinara sauce for dipping.

Servings: 4

Nutritional Information (per serving):

Calories: 180 kcal
Total Fat: 8g
Saturated Fat: 4g
Trans Fat: 0g
Cholesterol: 90mg
Sodium: 320mg
Total Carbohydrates: 10g
Dietary Fiber: 1g
Sugars: 1g
Protein: 15g

7.2 Irresistible Dips and Spreads for Entertaining

1. Classic Guacamole

Ingredients:

- 3 ripe avocados
- 1 small onion, finely diced
- 2 Roma tomatoes, diced
- 1 jalapeño pepper, seeded and minced
- 2 cloves garlic, minced
- Juice of 1 lime
- 1/4 cup fresh cilantro, chopped
- Salt and pepper to taste

Directions:

1. Remove the pits from the avocados, cut them in half, and scoop out the meat into a dish.
2. Using a fork, mash the avocados until smooth, adding more pieces if preferred.
3. Add the chopped cilantro, lime juice, minced garlic, minced jalapeño pepper, diced onion, and diced tomatoes and stir.
4. To taste, add salt and pepper for seasoning.
5. When ready to serve, either cover and chill or serve right away.

Servings: 6

Nutritional Information (per serving):

Calories: 160 kcal

Total Fat: 14g

Saturated Fat: 2g

Trans Fat: 0g

Cholesterol: 0mg

Sodium: 10mg

Total Carbohydrates: 10g

Dietary Fiber: 7g

Sugars: 1g

Protein: 2g

2. Spinach and Artichoke Dip

Ingredients:

- 1 (10 ounce) container of thawed and drained frozen chopped spinach
- One can (14 oz) of drained and diced artichoke hearts
- One cup shredded mozzarella cheese
- 1/2 cup grated Parmesan cheese
- 1/2 cup mayonnaise
- 1/2 cup sour cream
- 2 cloves garlic, minced
- Salt and pepper to taste

Directions:

1. Turn the oven on to 375°F, or 190°C.
2. Mix the chopped spinach, chopped artichoke hearts, grated Parmesan cheese, shredded mozzarella cheese, mayonnaise, sour cream, and minced garlic in a big bowl.
3. Toss to thoroughly mix in the salt and pepper, if desired.
4. Using a spatula, smooth the mixture's surface after transferring it to a baking dish.
5. Bake in the preheated oven for 25-30 minutes, or until the dip is bubbly and golden brown on top.
6. Serve hot with tortilla chips, crackers, or sliced baguette.

Servings: 8

Nutritional Information (per serving):

Calories: 250 kcal

Total Fat: 21g

Saturated Fat: 6g

Trans Fat: 0g

Cholesterol: 25mg

Sodium: 470mg

Total Carbohydrates: 7g

Dietary Fiber: 2g

Sugars: 2g

Protein: 9g

3. Hummus

Ingredients:

- 1 (15 oz) can chickpeas, drained and rinsed
- 2 cloves garlic, minced
- 1/4 cup tahini
- 1/4 cup lemon juice
- 2 tablespoons olive oil
- 1/2 teaspoon ground cumin
- Salt to taste
- Water (as needed for consistency)

Directions:

1. In a food processor, combine the drained chickpeas, minced garlic, tahini, lemon juice, olive oil, ground cumin, and a pinch of salt.
2. Add water as necessary to get the appropriate consistency after blending until smooth.
3. Taste and adjust seasoning if necessary, adding more salt or lemon juice if desired.
4. Transfer the hummus to a serving bowl, drizzle with a little extra olive oil, and garnish with a sprinkle of paprika or chopped parsley if desired.
5. Serve with pita bread, crackers, or sliced vegetables.

Servings: 8

Nutritional Information (per serving):

Calories: 140 kcal
Total Fat: 9g
Saturated Fat: 1g
Trans Fat: 0g
Cholesterol: 0mg
Sodium: 160mg
Total Carbohydrates: 12g
Dietary Fiber: 3g
Sugars: 1g
Protein: 4g

4. Roasted Red Pepper Dip

Ingredients:

- 1 (12 oz) jar roasted red peppers, drained
- 1/2 cup Greek yogurt
- 1/4 cup cream cheese
- 2 cloves garlic, minced
- 2 tablespoons olive oil
- 1 tablespoon lemon juice
- 1 teaspoon paprika
- Salt and pepper to taste
- For garnish, use fresh parsley (optional).

Directions:

1. In a food processor, combine the drained roasted red peppers, Greek yogurt, cream cheese, minced garlic, olive oil, lemon juice, paprika, salt, and pepper.
2. Blend until smooth and creamy.
3. Taste and adjust seasoning if necessary, adding more salt or lemon juice if desired.
4. Transfer the dip to a serving bowl, garnish with fresh parsley if desired.

5. Accompany with crackers, veggie sticks, or pita chips.

Servings: 6

Nutritional Information (per serving):

Calories: 90 kcal

Total Fat: 7g

Saturated Fat: 2g

Trans Fat: 0g

Cholesterol: 10mg

Sodium: 170mg

Total Carbohydrates: 5g

Dietary Fiber: 1g

Sugars: 2g

Protein: 2g

5. Black Bean Salsa

Ingredients:

- 1 can (15 oz) black beans, drained and rinsed
- 1 cup corn kernels (fresh, canned, or frozen)
- 1 cup diced tomatoes
- 1/2 cup diced red onion
- 1/4 cup chopped fresh cilantro
- Juice of 1 lime
- 1 jalapeño pepper, seeded and minced (optional)
- Salt and pepper to taste

Directions:

1. In a large bowl, combine the drained black beans, corn kernels, diced tomatoes, diced red onion, chopped fresh cilantro, minced jalapeño pepper (if using), and lime juice.
2. Season with salt and pepper to taste and toss until well combined.

3. Cover and refrigerate for at least 30 minutes to allow the flavors to meld.

4. Taste and adjust seasoning if necessary before serving.

5. Serve with tortilla chips or as a topping for grilled meats or fish.

Servings: 6

Nutritional Information (per serving):

Calories: 120 kcal

Total Fat: 0.5g

Saturated Fat: 0g

Trans Fat: 0g

Cholesterol: 0mg

Sodium: 290mg

Total Carbohydrates: 23g

Dietary Fiber: 6g

Sugars:

7.3 Quick and Easy Zero Point Appetizers

1. Cucumber Bites with Tzatziki

Ingredients:

- 1 large cucumber
- 1/2 cup plain non-fat Greek yogurt
- 1/4 cup grated cucumber
- 1 clove garlic, minced
- 1 tablespoon fresh dill, chopped
- 1 tablespoon lemon juice
- Salt and pepper to taste

Directions:

1. Slice the cucumber into rounds, about 1/4 inch thick.
2. In a small bowl, mix together Greek yogurt, grated cucumber, minced garlic, chopped dill, lemon juice, salt, and pepper.
3. Top each cucumber round with a dollop of tzatziki mixture.
4. Garnish with additional fresh dill if desired.
5. Serve chilled.

Servings: 4

Nutritional Information (per serving):

Calories: 20 kcal

Total Fat: 0g

Saturated Fat: 0g

Trans Fat: 0g

Cholesterol: 0mg

Sodium: 15mg

Total Carbohydrates: 3g

Dietary Fiber: 1g

Sugars: 1g

Protein: 3g

2. Bell Pepper Nachos

Ingredients:

- 2 large bell peppers (any color), halved and seeded
- 1/2 cup black beans, drained and rinsed
- 1/4 cup salsa
- 1/4 cup diced tomatoes
- 1/4 cup diced red onion
- 11/4 cup of reduced-fat cheddar cheese, shredded
- For garnish, fresh cilantro is optional.

Directions:

1. Turn the oven on to 375°F, or 190°C.
2. Place the bell pepper halves on a baking sheet lined with parchment paper.
3. Fill each bell pepper half with black beans, salsa, diced tomatoes, and diced red onion.
4. Top with shredded cheddar cheese.
5. Bake for 10 to 12 minutes, or until the cheese is bubbling and melted, in a preheated oven.
6. If desired, garnish with fresh cilantro.
7. Warm up the food.

Servings: 4

Nutritional Information (per serving):

Calories: 40 kcal

Total Fat: 0.5g

Saturated Fat: 0g

Trans Fat: 0g

Cholesterol: 0mg

Sodium: 150mg

Total Carbohydrates: 7g

Dietary Fiber: 2g

Sugars: 2g

Protein: 3g

3. Cucumber Sushi Rolls

Ingredients:

- 1 large cucumber
- 1/4 cup shredded carrots
- 1/4 cup shredded red cabbage
- 1/4 cup avocado slices
- Two teaspoons of soy sauce with lower sodium
- For serving, wasabi and pickled ginger are optional.

Directions:

1. Slice the cucumber lengthwise into thin strips using a vegetable peeler or mandoline slicer.
2. Lay the cucumber strips flat and place shredded carrots, shredded red cabbage, and avocado slices on top.
3. Roll up each cucumber strip tightly to form sushi rolls.
4. If necessary, fasten with toothpicks.
5. Serve with reduced-sodium soy sauce, wasabi, and pickled ginger on the side if desired.

Servings: 4

Nutritional Information (per serving):

Calories: 20 kcal

Total Fat: 1g

Saturated Fat: 0g

Trans Fat: 0g

Cholesterol: 0mg

Sodium: 140mg

Total Carbohydrates: 4g

Dietary Fiber: 1g

Sugars: 1g

Protein: 1g

4. Caprese Skewers

Ingredients:

- 8 cherry tomatoes
- 8 small fresh mozzarella balls (bocconcini)
- 8 fresh basil leaves
- Balsamic glaze for drizzling

Directions:

1. Thread one cherry tomato, one mozzarella ball, and one basil leaf onto each skewer.
2. Place the skewers on a dish for serving.
3. Drizzle with balsamic glaze just before serving.
4. Serve at room temperature.

Servings: 4

Nutritional Information (per serving):

Calories: 30 kcal

Total Fat: 2g

Saturated Fat: 1g

Trans Fat: 0g

Cholesterol: 5mg

Sodium: 20mg

Total Carbohydrates: 1g

Dietary Fiber: 0g

Sugars: 1g

Protein: 2g

5. Greek Salad Skewers

Ingredients:

- 8 cherry tomatoes
- 8 cucumber chunks
- 8 Kalamata olives
- 8 small cubes of feta cheese
- Fresh oregano for garnish (optional)
- Greek vinaigrette for drizzling

Directions:

1. Thread one cherry tomato, one cucumber chunk, one Kalamata olive, and one cube of feta cheese onto each skewer.
2. Arrange the skewers on a serving platter.
3. Drizzle with Greek vinaigrette just before serving.
4. Garnish with fresh oregano if desired.
5. Serve at room temperature.

Servings: 4

Nutritional Information (per serving):

Calories: 40 kcal

Total Fat: 3g

Saturated Fat: 1g

Trans Fat: 0g

Cholesterol: 5mg

Sodium: 120mg
Total Carbohydrates: 2g
Dietary Fiber: 1g
Sugars: 1g
Protein: 2g

Chapter 8: Sweet Treats Without the Guilt

8.1 Indulgent Desserts Made with Zero Point Ingredients

1. Mixed Berry Sorbet

Ingredients:

- 2 cups mixed berries (such as strawberries, blueberries, and raspberries), frozen
- 1/4 cup plain non-fat Greek yogurt
- 1 tablespoon lemon juice
- 1-2 tablespoons sweetener of choice (optional)

Directions:

1. In a blender or food processor, combine the frozen mixed berries, Greek yogurt, lemon juice, and sweetener (if using).
2. Blend until creamy and smooth, stopping occasionally to scrape down the edges of the food processor or blender.
3. Transfer the sorbet mixture to a shallow dish and freeze for 2-3 hours, or until firm.
4. Once firm, use a fork to scrape the sorbet to create a fluffy texture.
5. Serve immediately or store in the freezer until ready to serve.

2. Chocolate Banana "Nice Cream"

Ingredients:

- 2 ripe bananas, sliced and frozen
- Two tsp of cocoa powder without sugar added
- 1 tablespoon plain non-fat Greek yogurt
- 1 teaspoon vanilla extract

Directions:

1. In a blender or food processor, combine the frozen banana slices, cocoa powder, Greek yogurt, and vanilla extract.
2. Blend until smooth and creamy, scraping down the sides of the blender or food processor as needed.
3. Transfer the "nice cream" to a shallow dish and freeze for 1-2 hours, or until firm.
4. Serve immediately for a soft-serve texture, or let it sit at room temperature for a few minutes to soften slightly before serving.

3. Lemon Poppy Seed Frozen Yogurt

Ingredients:

- 2 cups plain non-fat Greek yogurt
- Zest and juice of 1 lemon
- 2 tablespoons sweetener of choice (such as honey or maple syrup)
- 1 tablespoon poppy seeds

Directions:

1. In a mixing bowl, combine the Greek yogurt, lemon zest, lemon juice, sweetener, and poppy seeds.
2. Stir until well combined.
3. Pour the mixture into an ice cream machine and churn until it reaches a soft-serve consistency, generally 20 to 25 minutes, depending on the manufacturer's specifications.
4. Serve immediately for a soft texture or transfer to a container and freeze for 1-2 hours for a firmer texture.
5. Enjoy as is or with additional lemon zest or poppy seeds sprinkled on top.

4. Pineapple Coconut Popsicles

Ingredients:

- 2 cups fresh pineapple chunks
- 1/2 cup light coconut milk
- 1 tablespoon sweetener of choice (optional)

Directions:

1. In a blender, combine the pineapple chunks, coconut milk, and sweetener (if using).
2. Blend till creamy and smooth.
3. Leaving a small amount of room at the top for expansion, pour the mixture into the popsicle molds.
4. Place popsicle sticks into every mold.
5. Freeze for at least 4-6 hours, or until completely firm.
6. To release the popsicles, run warm water over the outside of the molds for a few seconds.
7. Serve immediately and enjoy!

5. Berry Chia Seed Pudding

Ingredients:

- 1 cup unsweetened almond milk (or any milk of choice)
- 1/4 cup chia seeds
- 1/2 teaspoon vanilla extract
- Mixed berries for topping

Directions:

1. In a mixing bowl, whisk together the almond milk, chia seeds, and vanilla extract.
2. Cover and refrigerate for at least 2 hours, or overnight, until the mixture thickens and becomes pudding-like.
3. Once the chia pudding is ready, divide it into serving cups or bowls.
4. Top with fresh mixed berries just before serving.

Enjoy immediately or store in the refrigerator for up to 3 days.

These indulgent desserts made with zero point ingredients are perfect for satisfying your sweet tooth while staying on track with your healthy eating goals. Enjoy them guilt-free!

8.2 Healthy Baking Alternatives for a Sweet Tooth Fix

Banana Oatmeal Cookies:

Ingredients:

- 2 ripe bananas, mashed
- 1 cup rolled oats
- 1/4 cup raisins or chocolate chips (optional)
- 1/2 teaspoon cinnamon
- 1/4 teaspoon vanilla extract
- Directions:
- Adjust the oven temperature to 350°F (175°C) and place parchment paper on a baking pan.
- Mashed bananas, rolled oats, chocolate chips or raisins (if used), cinnamon, and vanilla essence should all be thoroughly mixed together in a dish.
- Spoon mixture onto baking sheet that has been prepared.
- Bake the cookies for 12 to 15 minutes, or until they turn golden brown.
- Let cool completely before serving.

Greek Yogurt Blueberry Muffins:

Ingredients:

- 1 cup whole wheat flour
- 1 cup rolled oats
- 1 teaspoon baking powder
- 1/2 teaspoon baking soda
- 1/4 teaspoon salt
- 1 cup plain Greek yogurt
- 1/4 cup honey or maple syrup
- 1/4 cup unsweetened applesauce
- 1 egg
- 1 teaspoon vanilla extract

- One cup fresh or frozen blueberries

Directions:

1. Heat the oven to 375°F (190°C) and place paper liners into a muffin tray.
2. Mix the flour, oats, baking soda, baking powder, and salt in a large basin.
3. Smoothly combine Greek yogurt, applesauce, egg, honey or maple syrup, and vanilla extract in a separate dish.
4. Mix until just mixed, pour the wet components into the dry ingredients.
5. Fold in the blueberries gently.
6. Evenly distribute the batter among the muffin cups.
7. When a toothpick put into the center comes out clean, bake for 18 to 20 minutes.
8. Let cool completely before serving.

Zucchini Brownies:

Ingredients:

- 1/4 cup of unsweetened applesauce and one cup of shredded zucchini with extra moisture squeezed out
- 1/4 cup maple syrup or honey
- One egg
- One tsp vanilla essence
- Half a cup of whole wheat flour
- 1/4 cup chocolate powder, unsweetened
- One-half tsp baking soda
- 1/4 tsp salt
- 1/4 cup dark chocolate chips (optional)

Directions:

1. Preheat the oven to 350°F (175°C) and grease an 8x8-inch baking pan.
2. Grated zucchini, applesauce, honey (or maple syrup), egg, and vanilla essence should all be thoroughly mixed together in a dish.
3. Mix the flour, baking soda, cocoa powder, and salt in a separate basin.
4. Stirring until just blended, gradually add the dry ingredients to the wet components.
5. If using, mix in the dark chocolate chips.
6. Evenly distribute the batter after pouring it into the baking pan.

7. When a toothpick put into the center comes out clean, bake for 25 to 30 minutes.

8. Let cool completely before slicing and serving.

Applesauce Oatmeal Bread:

Ingredients:
- 1 cup unsweetened applesauce
- 1/4 cup honey or maple syrup
- 1 egg
- 1 teaspoon vanilla extract
- 1 1/2 cups rolled oats
- 1/2 cup whole wheat flour
- 1 teaspoon baking powder
- 1/2 teaspoon baking soda
- 1/2 teaspoon cinnamon
- 1/4 teaspoon salt
- 1/2 cup chopped nuts or dried fruit (optional)

Directions:
1. Oil a loaf pan and preheat the oven to 350°F (175°C).
2. Applesauce, honey (or maple syrup), egg, and vanilla extract should all be well mixed together in a big basin.
3. Mix the oats, flour, baking soda, baking powder, cinnamon, and salt in a separate dish.
4. Stirring until just blended, gradually add the dry ingredients to the wet components.
5. If using, mix with chopped almonds or dried fruit.
6. After the loaf pan is ready, pour the batter into it.
7. When a toothpick put into the center comes out clean, bake for 35 to 40 minutes.
8. Let it cool down before cutting and serving.

Coconut Flour Pancakes:

Ingredients:
- 4 eggs
- 1/2 cup unsweetened almond milk (or any milk of choice)

- 1/4 cup coconut flour
- 1 tablespoon honey or maple syrup
- 1 teaspoon vanilla extract
- 1/2 teaspoon baking powder
- Pinch of salt
- Coconut oil for cooking

Directions:

1. In a bowl, whisk together eggs, almond milk, honey or maple syrup, and vanilla extract until well combined.
2. Add coconut flour, baking powder, and salt to the wet ingredients and whisk until smooth.
3. Let the batter sit for a few minutes to allow the coconut flour to absorb the liquid.
4. Heat a non-stick skillet or griddle over medium heat and lightly grease with coconut oil.
5. Pour about 1/4 cup of batter onto the skillet for each pancake.
6. Cook for 2-3 minutes, or until bubbles form on the surface, then flip and cook for another 1-2 minutes until golden brown.
7. Proceed with the leftover batter.
8. Serve warm with your favorite toppings such as fresh fruit, yogurt, or nut butter.

8.3 Decadent Frozen Treats for Any Season

Chocolate Dipped Frozen Banana Bites:

Ingredients:

- 2 ripe bananas, peeled and cut into thick slices
- 1/2 cup dark chocolate chips
- 1 tablespoon coconut oil
- Toppings of your choice (crushed nuts, shredded coconut, sprinkles)

Directions:

1. Place banana slices on a parchment-lined baking sheet and insert a toothpick into each slice.
2. Freeze the banana slices for at least 1 hour.
3. In a microwave-safe bowl, melt dark chocolate chips with coconut oil in 30-second intervals, stirring until smooth.
4. Dip each frozen banana slice into the melted chocolate, coating it completely.
5. Quickly sprinkle desired toppings over the chocolate before it hardens.
6. Return the coated banana slices to the parchment-lined baking sheet and freeze for an additional 30 minutes, or until the chocolate is set.
7. Serve right away or put in the freezer in an airtight container.

Peanut Butter and Jelly Frozen Yogurt Bites:

Ingredients:

- 1 cup plain Greek yogurt
- 2 tablespoons peanut butter
- 2 tablespoons raspberry or strawberry jam
- Directions:
- In a bowl, mix together Greek yogurt and peanut butter until smooth.
- Use small muffin liners to line a mini muffin tray.
- Spoon a small amount of the yogurt mixture into each muffin liner, filling them about halfway.

- Add a small dollop of jam on top of the yogurt in each muffin liner.
- Cover the jam with more yogurt mixture, filling the muffin liners to the top.
- Freeze the yogurt bites for at least 2 hours, or until firm.
- Once frozen, remove the yogurt bites from the muffin tin and store them in a freezer bag or container.
- Enjoy straight from the freezer as a refreshing snack.

Coconut Mango Popsicles:

Ingredients:
- 2 ripe mangoes, peeled and diced
- 1 cup coconut milk
- 2 tablespoons honey or maple syrup
- 1 teaspoon vanilla extract
- Directions:
- Place diced mangoes, coconut milk, honey or maple syrup, and vanilla extract in a blender.
- Blend till creamy and smooth.
- Fill up all of the popsicle molds with the mango mixture.
- Place a popsicle stick into every mold.
- The popsicles should be frozen for a minimum of 4 hours, or until fully firm.
- Run the popsicles under warm water for a short while to extract them from the molds.
- Savor the tastes of the tropics as soon as you serve!

Dark Chocolate Avocado Ice Cream:

Ingredients:
- Two ripe avocados, peeled and pitted
- 1/2 cup unsweetened cocoa powder
- 1/2 cup coconut milk
- 1/4 cup honey or maple syrup
- 1 teaspoon vanilla extract
- Pinch of salt

Directions:

1. Place avocados, cocoa powder, coconut milk, honey or maple syrup, vanilla extract, and salt in a blender.
2. Blend until smooth and creamy.
3. Pour the ingredients into an ice cream maker and process as directed by the manufacturer.
4. Once churned, transfer the ice cream to a freezer-safe container and freeze for an additional 2-3 hours, or until firm.
5. Serve scoops of the ice cream in bowls or cones and enjoy the rich, creamy texture.

Strawberry Cheesecake Frozen Yogurt Bites:

Ingredients:

- 1 cup plain Greek yogurt
- 2 tablespoons cream cheese, softened
- 2 tablespoons honey or maple syrup
- 1/2 cup diced strawberries
- Graham cracker crumbs for garnish (optional)

Directions:

1. In a bowl, mix together Greek yogurt, softened cream cheese, and honey or maple syrup until smooth.
2. Gently fold in diced strawberries.
3. Spoon the yogurt mixture into mini muffin liners or silicone molds.
4. Sprinkle graham cracker crumbs on top for added crunch (optional).
5. Freeze the yogurt bites for at least 2 hours, or until firm.

6. Once frozen, remove the yogurt bites from the molds and transfer them to a freezer bag or container.
7. Enjoy these creamy and fruity bites straight from the freezer whenever you crave a sweet treat!
8. These decadent frozen treats are perfect for satisfying your sweet cravings while providing a refreshing and healthier option. Enjoy experimenting with these recipes!

Chapter 9: Drinks to Quench Your Thirst

9.1 Refreshing Zero Point Beverages for Hydration

Cucumber Mint Infused Water:

Ingredients:

- 1 cucumber, sliced
- 10-12 fresh mint leaves
- Water

Directions:

1. Place cucumber slices and mint leaves in a pitcher.
2. Fill the pitcher with water.
3. Stir gently to combine.
4. Let the flavors steep for at least an hour by placing it in the refrigerator.
5. Serve over ice and enjoy this refreshing and hydrating drink.

Servings: 4

Nutritional Information (per serving):

Calories: 0 kcal

Total Fat: 0g

Sodium: 0mg

Total Carbohydrates: 0g

Sugars: 0g

Protein: 0g

Lemon Ginger Iced Tea:

Ingredients:

- 4 cups water
- 4 bags of your favorite tea (green, black, or herbal)
- 1 lemon, thinly sliced
- One-inch piece of fresh ginger, thinly sliced

Directions:

1. Heat the water in a pot until it boils.
2. After turning off the heat, add the tea bags, ginger, and lemon segments.
3. Steep for five to seven minutes.
4. After removing the tea bags, let the mixture reach room temperature.
5. Pour into a pitcher and chill in the fridge.
6. Serve over ice and garnish with extra lemon slices if desired.

Servings: 4

Nutritional Information (per serving):

Calories: 0 kcal

Total Fat: 0g

Sodium: 0mg

Total Carbohydrates: 0g

Sugars: 0g

Protein: 0g

Watermelon Lime Cooler:

Ingredients:

- 2 cups cubed seedless watermelon
- Juice of 2 limes
- 2 cups cold water
- Ice cubes

Directions:

1. In a blender, combine watermelon cubes and lime juice.
2. Blend until smooth.
3. To get rid of any pulp, strain the mixture using a fine mesh screen.
4. Transfer the strained juice to a pitcher and add cold water.
5. Stir to combine.
6. Serve over ice and garnish with lime slices if desired.

Servings: 4

Nutritional Information (per serving):

Calories: 15 kcal

Total Fat: 0g

Sodium: 0mg

Total Carbohydrates: 4g

Sugars: 3g

Protein: 0g

Berry Citrus Sparkling Water:

Ingredients:

- 1 cup mixed berries (strawberries, blueberries, raspberries)
- Juice of 1 lemon
- Juice of 1 orange
- 4 cups sparkling water
- Ice cubes

Directions:

1. In a blender, puree mixed berries, lemon juice, and orange juice until smooth.
2. Strain the mixture through a fine mesh sieve to remove any seeds.
3. Divide the berry citrus puree among four glasses filled with ice cubes.
4. Top each glass with sparkling water.
5. Stir gently to combine.
6. Garnish with extra berries or citrus slices if desired.

Servings: 4

Nutritional Information (per serving):

Calories: 10 kcal

Total Fat: 0g

Sodium: 0mg

Total Carbohydrates: 3g

Sugars: 1g

Protein: 0g

Minty Pineapple Coconut Water:

Ingredients:

- 2 cups coconut water
- 1 cup fresh pineapple chunks
- 1/4 cup fresh mint leaves
- Ice cubes

Directions:

1. In a blender, combine coconut water, pineapple chunks, and mint leaves.
2. Blend until smooth.
3. Strain the mixture through a fine mesh sieve to remove any pulp.
4. Transfer the strained juice to a pitcher.
5. Chill in the refrigerator for at least 30 minutes.
6. Serve over ice and garnish with mint leaves if desired.

Servings: 4

Nutritional Information (per serving):

Calories: 20 kcal

Total Fat: 0g

Sodium: 25mg

Total Carbohydrates: 5g

Sugars: 3g

Protein: 0g

These refreshing zero point beverages are perfect for staying hydrated while enjoying delicious flavors. Feel free to adjust the ingredients and quantities to suit your taste preferences. Enjoy!

9.2 Creative Mocktails and Infusions for Flavor

Virgin Mojito Mocktail:

Ingredients:

- 1/2 lime, cut into wedges
- 8-10 fresh mint leaves
- 1 tablespoon sugar (optional)
- 1 cup club soda
- Ice cubes

Directions:

1. In a glass, muddle together lime wedges, mint leaves, and sugar (if using) until fragrant.
2. Fill the glass with ice cubes.
3. Pour club soda over the ice.
4. Stir gently to combine.
5. Add a lime slice and a mint sprig as garnish.
6. Serving: 1 mocktail

Nutritional Information:

Calories: 10 kcal

Total Fat: 0g

Sodium: 40mg

Total Carbohydrates: 3g

Sugars: 1g

Protein: 0g

Berry Basil Spritzer:

Ingredients:

- 1/2 cup mixed berries (strawberries, blueberries, raspberries)
- 2-3 fresh basil leaves
- 1 tablespoon honey or agave syrup
- 1 cup sparkling water

- Ice cubes

Directions:

1. In a glass, muddle together mixed berries, basil leaves, and honey or agave syrup until well combined.
2. Place ice cubes in the glass.
3. Pour sparkling water over the ice.
4. Stir gently to combine.
5. Garnish with a few whole berries and a basil leaf.
6. Serving: 1 mocktail

Nutritional Information:

Calories: 30 kcal

Total Fat: 0g

Sodium: 0mg

Total Carbohydrates: 8g

Sugars: 7g

Protein: 0g

Cucumber Lavender Lemonade:

Ingredients:

- 1/2 cucumber, sliced
- 1 tablespoon dried culinary lavender
- 1/4 cup honey or maple syrup
- Juice of 2 lemons
- 3 cups cold water
- Ice cubes

Directions:

1. In a pitcher, combine cucumber slices, dried lavender, honey or maple syrup, lemon juice, and cold water.
2. To dissolve the sweetener, thoroughly stir.
3. Let the flavors steep for at least an hour by placing it in the refrigerator.
4. Pour the contents into serving glasses with ice cubes after straining through a fine mesh screen.

5. Add a piece of cucumber or a touch of lemon as garnish.

Serving: 1 mocktail

Nutritional Information:

Calories: 60 kcal

Total Fat: 0g

Sodium: 0mg

Total Carbohydrates: 17g

Sugars: 15g

Protein: 0g

Pineapple Ginger Agua Fresca:

Ingredients:

- 1 cup fresh pineapple chunks
- 1-inch piece of fresh ginger, peeled and sliced
- 2 cups cold water
- 1 tablespoon honey or agave syrup
- Ice cubes

Directions:

1. In a blender, combine pineapple chunks, fresh ginger slices, cold water, and honey or agave syrup.
2. Blend until smooth.
3. Strain the mixture through a fine mesh sieve into a pitcher.
4. Chill in the refrigerator for at least 30 minutes.
5. Pour the agua fresca into serving glasses filled with ice cubes.
6. Garnish with a pineapple wedge or a slice of ginger.

Serving: 1 mocktail

Nutritional Information:

Calories: 50 kcal

Total Fat: 0g

Sodium: 0mg

Total Carbohydrates: 13g

Sugars: 10g

Protein: 0g

Citrus Rosemary Spritz:

Ingredients:
- 1/2 orange, sliced
- 1/2 lemon, sliced
- 2-3 sprigs of fresh rosemary
- 1 tablespoon honey or agave syrup
- 1 cup sparkling water
- Ice cubes

Directions:
1. In a glass, muddle together orange slices, lemon slices, rosemary sprigs, and honey or agave syrup until fragrant.
2. Fill the glass with ice cubes.
3. Pour sparkling water over the ice.
4. Stir gently to combine.
5. Garnish with a citrus twist and a fresh rosemary sprig.

Serving: 1 mocktail

Nutritional Information:

Calories: 30 kcal

Total Fat: 0g

Sodium: 0mg

Total Carbohydrates: 8g

Sugars: 7g

Protein: 0g

These creative mocktails and infusions offer delicious flavors and are perfect for any occasion. Enjoy them as refreshing alternatives to alcoholic beverages while staying hydrated! Adjust sweeteners and ingredients according to your taste preferences.

9.3 Energizing Smoothies and Shakes

Green Power Smoothie:

Ingredients:
- 1 cup spinach
- 1/2 ripe banana
- 1/2 cup pineapple chunks
- 1/2 cup mango chunks
- 1/2 cup unsweetened almond milk
- 1 tablespoon chia seeds

Directions:
1. Place spinach, banana, pineapple chunks, mango chunks, almond milk, and chia seeds in a blender.
2. Blend until smooth and creamy.
3. Pour into a glass and enjoy immediately.

Servings: 1

Nutritional Information (per serving):

Calories: 250 kcal

Total Fat: 6g

Saturated Fat: 0.5g

Trans Fat: 0g

Cholesterol: 0mg

Sodium: 120mg

Total Carbohydrates: 47g

Dietary Fiber: 11g

Sugars: 27g

Protein: 6g

Berry Blast Protein Smoothie:

Ingredients:

- 1/2 cup mixed berries (strawberries, blueberries, raspberries)
- 1/2 ripe banana
- One and half cup plain Greek yogurt
- One and half cup unsweetened almond milk
- 1 scoop vanilla protein powder
- 1 tablespoon honey or maple syrup (optional)

Directions:

1. Place mixed berries, banana, Greek yogurt, almond milk, protein powder, and honey or maple syrup (if using) in a blender.
2. Blend until smooth and well combined.
3. Pour into a glass and start sipping right away.

Servings: 1

Nutritional Information (per serving):

Calories: 290 kcal

Total Fat: 3g

Saturated Fat: 0g

Trans Fat: 0g

Cholesterol: 10mg

Sodium: 180mg

Total Carbohydrates: 41g

Dietary Fiber: 7g

Sugars: 26g

Protein: 27g

Tropical Turmeric Smoothie:

Ingredients:

- 1/2 cup frozen pineapple chunks
- 1/2 cup frozen mango chunks
- 1 small banana

- 1/2 teaspoon ground turmeric
- 1/2 teaspoon ground ginger
- 1 cup coconut water

Directions:

1. Place frozen pineapple chunks, frozen mango chunks, banana, ground turmeric, ground ginger, and coconut water in a blender.
2. Blend until smooth and creamy.
3. Pour into a glass and enjoy immediately.

Servings: 1

Nutritional Information (per serving):

Calories: 280 kcal

Total Fat: 1g

Saturated Fat: 0g

Trans Fat: 0g

Cholesterol: 0mg

Sodium: 140mg

Total Carbohydrates: 68g

Dietary Fiber: 8g

Sugars: 45g

Protein: 4g

Peanut Butter Banana Protein Shake:

Ingredients:

- 1 ripe banana
- 2 tablespoons natural peanut butter
- One cup unsweetened almond milk
- 1 scoop chocolate protein powder
- 1/2 cup ice cubes

Directions:

1. Place ripe banana, peanut butter, almond milk, protein powder, and ice cubes in a blender.
2. Blend until smooth and creamy.

3. Pour into a glass and enjoy immediately.

Servings: 1

Nutritional Information (per serving):

Calories: 380 kcal

Total Fat: 16g

Saturated Fat: 2g

Trans Fat: 0g

Cholesterol: 25mg

Sodium: 280mg

Total Carbohydrates: 34g

Dietary Fiber: 7g

Sugars: 15g

Protein: 30g

Coffee Almond Protein Shake:

Ingredients:

- One and half cup brewed coffee, cooled
- One and half cup unsweetened almond milk
- 1 scoop vanilla or chocolate protein powder
- 1 tablespoon almond butter
- 1/2 teaspoon vanilla extract
- 1/2 teaspoon cinnamon (optional)
- 1/2 cup ice cubes

Directions:

1. In a blender, combine brewed coffee, almond milk, protein powder, almond butter, vanilla extract, cinnamon (if using), and ice cubes.
2. Blend until smooth and well combined.
3. Pour into a glass and enjoy immediately.

Servings: 1

Nutritional Information (per serving):

Calories: 250 kcal

Total Fat: 8g

Saturated Fat: 1g

Trans Fat: 0g

Cholesterol: 25mg

Sodium: 270mg

Total Carbohydrates: 10g

Dietary Fiber: 3g

Sugars: 3g

Protein: 30g

These energizing smoothies and shakes are packed with nutritious ingredients to fuel your day. Enjoy them as a delicious and convenient breakfast or snack option! Adjust ingredients and serving sizes as needed to fit your dietary preferences and requirements.

Chapter 10: Tips for Success and Sustainability

10.1 Staying Motivated on Your Zero Point Journey

Staying motivated on your zero point journey can be challenging at times, but with the right mindset and strategies, you can stay on track and achieve your goals. Here are a few hints to assist you with remaining persuaded:

1. Set Clear and Achievable Goals: Define specific and realistic goals for yourself on your zero point journey. Whether it's losing a certain amount of weight, improving your overall health, or fitting into a certain clothing size, having clear objectives will give you something to work towards and keep you focused.

2. Track Your Progress: Keep track of your progress regularly to see how far you've come. Whether you use a journal, a mobile app, or a tracking system provided by your weight loss program, seeing your accomplishments can be incredibly motivating and help you stay committed to your journey.

3. Celebrate Small Victories: Acknowledge and celebrate every achievement along the way, no matter how small. Whether it's losing a pound, sticking to your zero point meals for a week straight, or resisting temptation at a social gathering, pat yourself on the back and reward yourself for your efforts.

4. Stay Positive and Practice Self-Compassion: Focus on positive thinking and be kind to yourself throughout your journey. Understand that setbacks and challenges are a natural part of the process, and instead of beating yourself up over them, use them as opportunities to learn and grow. Practice self-compassion and treat yourself with the same kindness and understanding you would offer to a friend.

5. Find Support and Accountability: Surround yourself with a supportive network of friends, family, or fellow members of your weight loss program who can encourage and motivate you along the way. Share your successes, challenges, and goals with them, and lean on them for

support when you need it most. Having someone to hold you accountable can help keep you motivated and accountable.

6. Mix Things Up: Keep your zero point journey exciting and enjoyable by experimenting with new recipes, trying different types of exercise, or incorporating new healthy habits into your routine. Variety can help prevent boredom and keep you engaged and motivated to continue making progress.

7. Visualize Your Success: Take some time each day to visualize yourself achieving your goals and living the life you desire. Imagine how you will look, feel, and act when you reach your ideal weight and health. Visualizing success can help you stay motivated and focused on your journey, even when faced with challenges.

8. Practice Patience and Persistence: Remember that lasting change takes time, and progress may not always happen as quickly as you'd like. Be patient with yourself and trust in the process. Stay persistent, stay focused, and keep moving forward, one step at a time.

By incorporating these strategies into your zero point journey, you can stay motivated, overcome obstacles, and ultimately achieve success in reaching your health and wellness goals. Remember to stay focused on your why, stay positive, and celebrate every step of the way. You've got this!

10.2 Overcoming Challenges and Plateaus

Overcoming challenges and plateaus is an inevitable part of any journey towards achieving your health and wellness goals, including on a zero point diet. Here are some strategies to help you navigate and overcome these obstacles:

1. Identify the Problem: When facing a challenge or plateau, take some time to identify the root cause. Is it a lack of motivation, emotional eating, stress, or maybe you've hit a weight loss plateau? Understanding the underlying issue will help you address it more effectively.

2. Reevaluate Your Goals: Take a step back and reassess your goals. Are they still practical and reachable? Are they still motivating you? It's okay to adjust your goals as you progress on your journey to better align with your current circumstances and priorities.

3. Mix Up Your Routine: If you've hit a plateau in your weight loss or fitness journey, try mixing up your routine. Incorporate new exercises, try different zero point recipes, or change the intensity of your workouts. Adding variety can challenge your body in new ways and help break through the plateau.

4. Practice Mindful Eating: Be mindful of your eating habits and the reasons behind them. Are you eating out of hunger or emotions? Practice mindful eating by paying attention to your hunger cues, eating slowly, and savoring each bite. This can help prevent overeating and emotional eating.

5. Stay Consistent: Consistency is key to overcoming challenges and plateaus. Stay committed to your zero point journey, even when faced with setbacks or obstacles. Remember that progress takes time, and small, consistent efforts add up over time.

6. Seek Support: Don't be afraid to reach out for support when needed. Whether it's from friends, family, or a support group, having a support system can provide encouragement, accountability, and motivation during challenging times.

7. Focus on Non-Scale Victories: Shift your focus away from the scale and celebrate non-scale victories instead. Maybe you've noticed improvements in your energy levels, sleep quality, or overall mood. Celebrate these achievements as they indicate progress towards a healthier lifestyle.

8. Practice Self-Compassion: Be thoughtful to yourself during testing times. Understand that setbacks and plateaus are a natural part of the journey, and it's okay to experience them. Practice self-compassion by treating yourself with understanding, patience, and forgiveness.

9. Stay Patient and Persistent: Overcoming challenges and plateaus requires patience and persistence. Stay committed to your goals, trust in the process, and keep moving forward, one step at a time. Remember that setbacks are temporary, and with perseverance, you can overcome them.

10. Celebrate Your Progress: Take time to celebrate your progress and achievements along the way, no matter how small. Acknowledge the hard work and effort you've put in and use it as motivation to keep pushing forward towards your goals.

By implementing these strategies, you can overcome challenges and plateaus on your zero point journey and continue making progress towards a healthier and happier lifestyle. Remember to stay positive, stay focused, and never give up on yourself. You're capable of achieving your goals!

10.3 Incorporating Zero Point Recipes into Your Lifestyle Long-Term

Incorporating zero point recipes into your lifestyle long-term can be a sustainable and effective way to maintain a healthy eating pattern while enjoying delicious and satisfying meals. Here are some tips for successfully integrating zero point recipes into your everyday life:

1. Gradual Transition: Start by gradually incorporating zero point recipes into your meal rotation. Begin with one or two recipes per week and gradually increase as you become more comfortable with them. This gradual approach allows you to adjust to the new eating habits without feeling overwhelmed.

2. Experiment with Variety: Explore a wide range of zero point recipes to keep your meals interesting and enjoyable. Try different cuisines, cooking methods, and flavor combinations to prevent boredom and maintain excitement about your meals.

3. Meal Planning and Preparation: Plan your meals ahead of time to ensure that you have the necessary ingredients on hand and to avoid the temptation of resorting to less healthy options. Set aside time each week for meal prep, including chopping vegetables, cooking grains, and preparing sauces or dressings, to streamline the cooking process during busy days.

4. Flexibility and Adaptability: Be flexible and adaptable with your zero point recipes to accommodate your preferences, dietary restrictions, and seasonal availability of ingredients. Feel free to modify recipes by adding or substituting ingredients to suit your taste and nutritional needs.

5. Portion Control: While zero point foods are low in calories and can be enjoyed freely, it's still important to practice portion control to ensure that you're not overeating. Pay attention to your hunger cues and stop eating when you feel satisfied, rather than when you're overly full.

6. Mindful Eating: Practice mindful eating by savoring each bite, chewing slowly, and paying attention to the flavors, textures, and sensations of the food. Eating mindfully can help you enjoy your meals more fully and prevent overeating.

7. Listen to Your Body: Tune into your body's signals of hunger and fullness and honor them accordingly. Eat when you're hungry and stop when you're satisfied, rather than relying on external cues or strict rules about when and how much to eat.

8. Stay Hydrated: Drink plenty of water throughout the day to stay hydrated and support your overall health and well-being. Opt for water or other zero calorie beverages to quench your thirst and prevent dehydration.

9. Practice Moderation: While zero point recipes can be a nutritious and satisfying part of your diet, it's important to practice moderation and balance with other food groups. Incorporate a variety of foods from all food groups to ensure that you're meeting your nutritional needs.

10. Enjoyment and Satisfaction: Above all, focus on enjoying your meals and finding satisfaction in the foods you eat. Choose zero point recipes that you genuinely enjoy and look forward to eating, and don't be afraid to indulge in occasional treats or indulgences in moderation.

By following these tips, you can successfully incorporate zero point recipes into your lifestyle long-term and enjoy the benefits of a balanced and nutritious diet. Remember to be patient with yourself, stay flexible, and celebrate your progress along the way.

Conclusion

In conclusion, "The Complete Zero Point Recipes for Weight Loss" offers a comprehensive guide to incorporating nutritious, flavorful, and satisfying meals into your weight loss journey. Throughout this book, we've explored a wide variety of zero point recipes that are not only delicious but also conducive to achieving your health and wellness goals.

From energizing breakfast smoothies to hearty soups, refreshing salads, flavorful entrees, and indulgent desserts, these recipes provide ample options to suit every palate and dietary preference. By focusing on whole, nutrient-dense ingredients and incorporating zero point foods, you can fuel your body with the nourishment it needs while still enjoying delicious meals that support your weight loss efforts.

In addition to providing a diverse array of recipes, this book has also offered valuable insights and tips for navigating challenges, staying motivated, and incorporating zero point recipes into your lifestyle long-term. By embracing mindful eating, practicing portion control, staying hydrated, and finding joy in the foods you eat, you can cultivate a sustainable approach to healthy eating that lasts a lifetime.

Remember, achieving and maintaining a healthy weight is not just about following a strict diet—it's about adopting a balanced and sustainable approach to eating that nourishes your body, mind, and soul. Whether you're just beginning your weight loss journey or you're looking for fresh inspiration to keep you on track, "The Complete Zero Point Recipes for Weight Loss" is here to support you every step of the way.

As you embark on this journey, I encourage you to approach it with patience, self-compassion, and an open mind. Embrace the process, celebrate your successes, and learn from your challenges. And above all, remember that you are capable of achieving your goals and living a vibrant, healthy life.

Thank you for joining me on this culinary adventure. Here's to your health, happiness, and success on your weight loss journey!